JUICING RECIPES *for* WEIGHT LOSS

Copyright © 2024 by Clara Levine

***

Table of Content

Introduction

Are you ready to embark on a transformative journey toward a healthier, leaner, and more energized you? Imagine sipping your way to a lighter, more vibrant self without sacrificing taste or spending hours in the kitchen. **Juicing Recipes for Weight Loss: Quick and Easy Juice Making Guide to Detox, Energize, Melt Fat, and Stay Fit** is here to help you achieve precisely that.

Finding the right balance between nutrition and convenience can be overwhelming in today's fast-paced world. We all want to lose weight, detox our bodies, and boost our energy levels, but knowing where to begin can be difficult. That is why this guide offers simple yet powerful solutions—nutrient-packed juices that can be made in minutes, fit into your busy lifestyle and deliver real results.

Whether your goal is to shed those extra pounds, enhance your overall health, or simply feel more energized throughout the day, these user-friendly juice recipes are tailored to your needs. From detoxifying greens to metabolism-boosting fruits, each recipe is meticulously designed to assist you in achieving your weight loss and wellness objectives.

So why wait? Take the first step towards a healthier, more energetic you today. By incorporating these delicious, fat-melting juices into your daily routine, you can kickstart your metabolism, cleanse your body, and feel rejuvenated in no time.

Are you prepared to transform your health and shed those extra pounds easily? Let's get started with juicing! You have the power to improve your health and vitality.

***

What is Juicing?

Juicing is the process of extracting liquid from fruits and vegetables, leaving behind the pulp primarily containing fiber. From a nutritional perspective, juicing offers a concentrated form of vitamins, minerals, and phytonutrients, making it an efficient way to consume various nutrients in a single serving. While it does not replace whole fruits and vegetables, juicing can complement a healthy diet by boosting nutrient intake.

The Nutritional Theory Behind Juicing

At its core, juicing delivers nutrients directly into the body, providing an immediate boost in energy, immune support, and overall wellness. This is especially appealing to those on detox programs or focusing on weight loss, as the body can quickly absorb these vitamins, minerals, and antioxidants without the fiber from whole produce.

For instance, vegetables like kale, spinach, and carrots are rich in vitamins A, C, and K and minerals like calcium, iron, and magnesium. Fruits such as oranges, berries, and apples offer potent antioxidants like vitamin C, reducing inflammation and supporting immune health. Juicing these foods together provides a fast, efficient way to meet daily nutrient needs.

Juicing for Weight Loss: The Science Explained

Juicing is a powerful tool for weight loss, thanks to its ability to provide nutrient-dense, low-calorie beverages. By replacing high-calorie, processed foods or sugary drinks with freshly made juices, many people experience a reduction in overall calorie intake, leading to gradual weight loss. The theory suggests that consuming these nutrient-packed juices helps satisfy the body's nutritional needs, curbing cravings for less healthy foods.

Certain ingredients are particularly beneficial for weight loss. For example, leafy greens, ginger, lemon, and cucumber are known for their detoxifying properties. They help flush out toxins, reduce water retention, and support metabolic function. Juices high in antioxidants and anti-inflammatory compounds may also improve digestion and fat metabolism.

Limitations and Considerations

While juicing is undeniably beneficial, it is important to approach it with balance. The fiber removed during the juicing process is essential for digestive health, blood sugar regulation, and feeling full. Therefore, it is crucial to incorporate whole fruits, vegetables, and other fiber-rich foods into your diet to maintain a balanced nutritional profile. This ensures that you can enjoy the benefits of juicing without compromising your overall health.

In conclusion, juicing offers a convenient way to increase nutrient intake, support weight loss, and boost energy, but it should be part of a comprehensive, well-rounded diet that includes whole foods.

Benefits of Juicing Versus Eating Raw Fruits and Vegetables

Juicing and eating raw fruits and vegetables both offer unique health benefits. Each method has advantages, and understanding them can help you make informed choices based on your dietary goals.

Benefits of Juicing

Quick Nutrient Absorption: Juicing removes fiber from fruits and vegetables, which means your body can more quickly absorb the vitamins, minerals, and antioxidants. This can provide an immediate boost in energy and nutrients, making it a convenient option for people looking to increase their intake of specific nutrients, especially during detoxes or fasts.

Concentrated Nutrient Intake: By juicing, you can consume more fruits and vegetables in one serving than eating them whole. For example, you may drink juice made from several fruits and vegetables that you need help eating all at once. This allows for a concentrated intake of vitamins, minerals, and phytonutrients.

Easy Digestion: Because the fiber is removed in the juicing process, the body can easily digest and assimilate the nutrients. For people with digestive issues or those recovering from illness, juicing can provide essential nutrients without overburdening the digestive system.

Hydration: Juicing offers a high water content, which supports hydration. Many fruits and vegetables, like cucumbers, celery, and watermelon, have high water levels that help maintain fluid balance.

Customizable Nutrient Profiles: Juicing allows mixing and matching fruits, vegetables, and herbs to create nutrient-dense blends tailored to your health goals. You can add ginger for inflammation, greens for detoxification, or lemon for immune support.

Benefits of Eating Raw Fruits and Vegetables

Retained Fiber Content: Whole fruits and vegetables benefit from their natural fiber content, which is crucial for digestive health, stabilizing blood sugar levels, and maintaining a healthy weight. Fiber helps slow the absorption of sugars, preventing rapid spikes in blood sugar and keeping you fuller for longer.

Sustained Energy: The fiber in raw fruits and vegetables helps with slow energy release. This provides more sustained energy than the quick nutrient surge from juice, which may lead to short-lived energy boosts followed by dips.

Balanced Nutrient Delivery: Whole fruits and vegetables provide a more balanced nutrient delivery. When you eat them raw, you get the vitamins and minerals, fiber, enzymes, and phytonutrients in their natural ratios, supporting overall gut health and digestion.

Fuller Feeling and Appetite Control: Chewing and consuming whole fruits and vegetables helps signal satiety to the brain, helping control portion sizes and reduce overeating. The fiber content also makes you feel fuller, making it easier to manage weight in the long term.

Lower Sugar Impact: Eating whole fruits is generally better for controlling blood sugar because fiber slows the digestion of sugars. This makes it less likely that you'll experience blood sugar spikes compared to consuming juices, which are often more concentrated in sugar, especially if made primarily from fruits.

In conclusion, juicing and eating raw fruits and vegetables offer valuable health benefits but serve different purposes. Juicing is excellent for quickly delivering nutrients and hydration in a concentrated form, while eating whole fruits and vegetables ensures a slower, more balanced nutrient intake with the added benefits of fiber. Ideally, a balanced diet would include both methods to maximize the benefits of each.

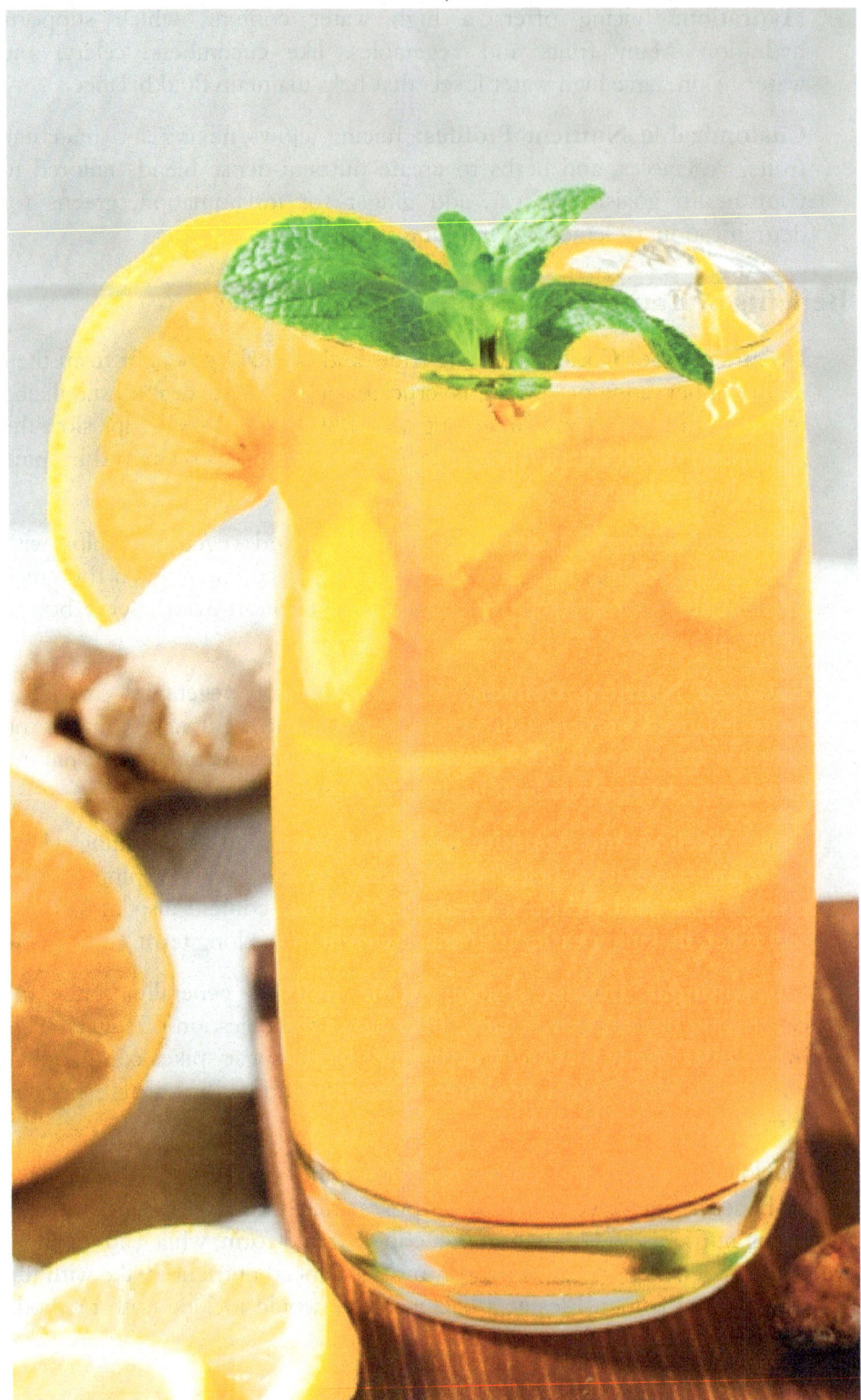

Healthy Morning Juices

Ginger and Turmeric Lemonade

Ginger and Turmeric Lemonade is a refreshing and healthy beverage that combines the potent benefits of turmeric, ginger, and lemon to create a potent immunity-boosting drink. This vibrant juice is perfect for weight loss, reducing inflammation, and detoxifying your body.

Servings: 2

Cook Time: 0 minutes

Prepping Time: 10 minutes

Difficulty: Easy

Ingredients:

- ✓ 1-inch fresh ginger, peeled and chopped
- ✓ 1 tsp turmeric powder (or 1-inch fresh turmeric root)
- ✓ 2 lemons, juiced
- ✓ 2 cups water
- ✓ 1 tbsp honey or maple syrup (optional)
- ✓ Pinch of black pepper

Step-by-Step Preparation:

1. Add the ginger, turmeric, and lemon juice to a blender.
2. Pour in the water and blend until smooth.
3. Strain the mixture to remove pulp, if desired.
4. Stir in honey or maple syrup for sweetness and a pinch of black pepper to enhance turmeric absorption.
5. Serve chilled over ice or as is.

Nutritional Facts: (Per serving)

- ❖ **Calories:** 40
- ❖ **Vitamin C:** 60% of RDA
- ❖ **Anti-inflammatory agents:** High
- ❖ **Detoxifying properties:** Excellent

This Ginger and Turmeric Lemonade is delicious and a fantastic way to support your body's natural detox processes and immunity. Enjoy this revitalizing drink daily for optimal weight management and overall wellness results.

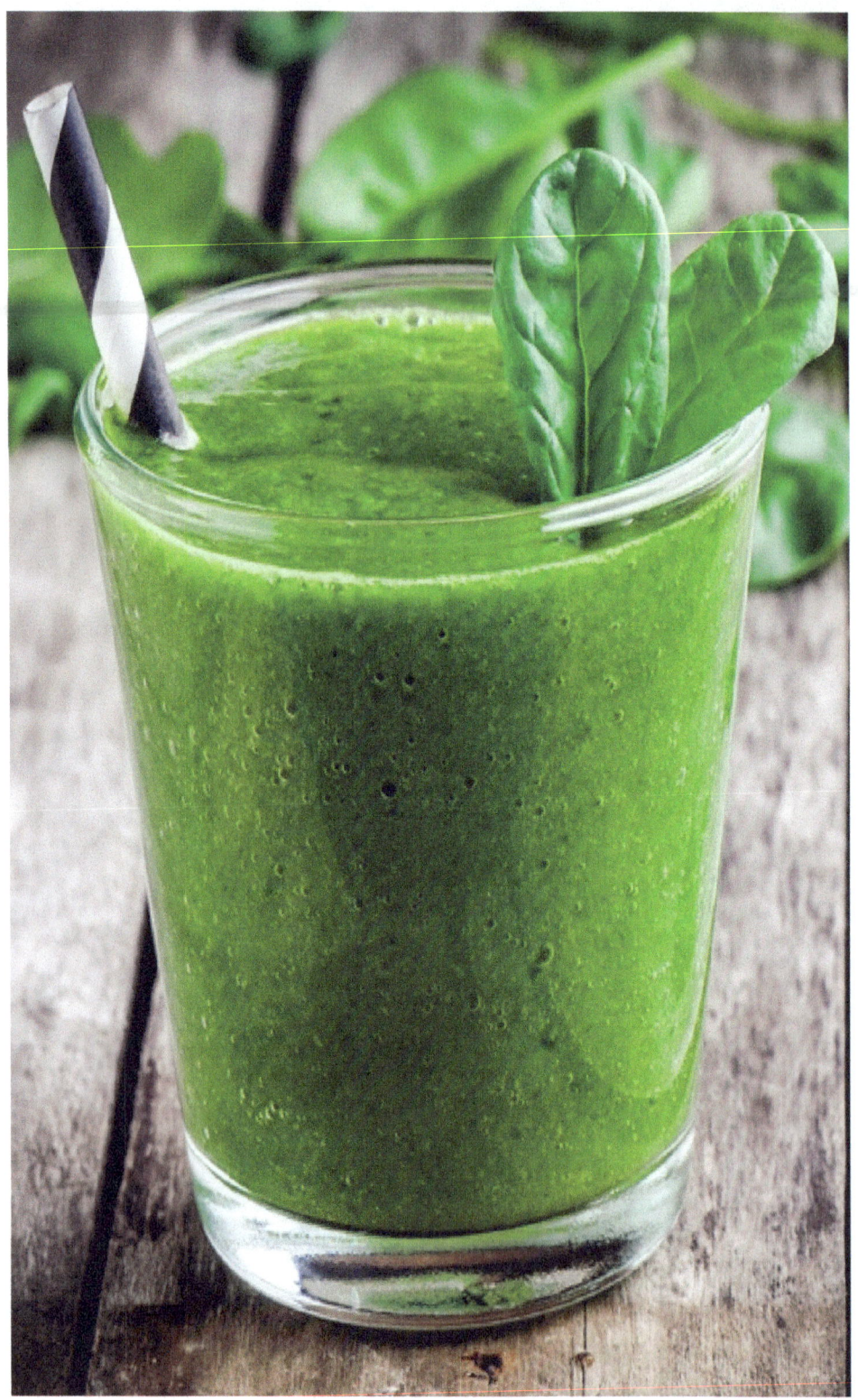

Green Spinach Smoothie

Green Spinach Smoothie is a nutrient-packed, refreshing drink designed to boost your metabolism and support weight loss. Loaded with spinach, fruits, and fiber, this smoothie helps you start your day on a healthy note while keeping you full and energized.

Servings: 1

Cook Time: 0 minutes

Prepping Time: 5 minutes

Difficulty: Easy

Ingredients:

- ✓ 1 cup fresh spinach
- ✓ 1/2 banana
- ✓ 1/2 green apple, chopped
- ✓ 1/2 cup almond milk (or water)
- ✓ 1 tbsp chia seeds
- ✓ 1/2 tsp fresh lemon juice

Step-by-Step Preparation:

1. Add spinach, banana, green apple, and almond milk (or water) to a blender.
2. Blend until smooth and creamy.
3. Add chia seeds and lemon juice, and blend again.
4. Pour into a glass and enjoy immediately.

Nutritional Facts: (Per serving)

- ❖ **Calories:** 120
- ❖ **Fiber:** 6g
- ❖ **Protein:** 3g
- ❖ **Vitamin A:** 60% of RDA
- ❖ **Vitamin C:** 40% of RDA

This Green Spinach Smoothie provides essential nutrients, keeps you feeling full, and supports weight loss efforts. Enjoy it as a refreshing breakfast or post-workout snack to fuel your body while keeping your calories in check.

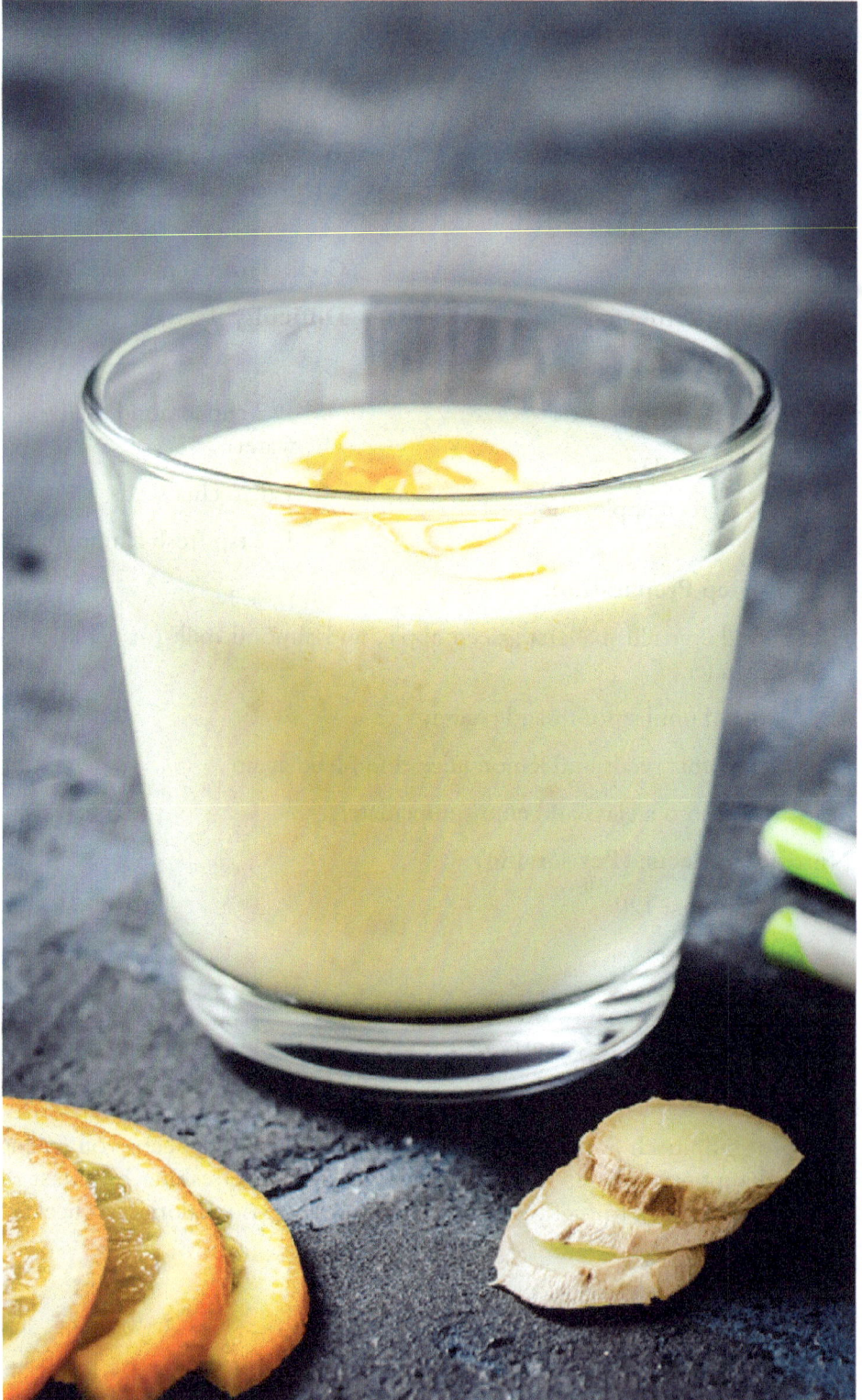

Turmeric, Orange Ginger Smoothie

Turmeric, Orange Ginger Smoothie is a zesty, anti-inflammatory drink packed with the power of turmeric, fresh oranges, and ginger. This smoothie boosts your metabolism, aids digestion, and helps with weight loss, making it a perfect addition to your daily routine.

Servings: 2

Cook Time: 0 minutes

Prepping Time: 5 minutes

Difficulty: Easy

Ingredients:

- ✓ 2 oranges, peeled and segmented
- ✓ 1-inch fresh ginger, peeled
- ✓ 1/2 tsp turmeric powder (or fresh turmeric)
- ✓ 1/2 cup coconut water
- ✓ 1 tsp honey (optional)
- ✓ Pinch of black pepper

Step-by-Step Preparation:

1. Add oranges, ginger, turmeric, and coconut water to a blender.
2. Blend until smooth.
3. Stir in honey for sweetness and a pinch of black pepper to enhance turmeric absorption.
4. Pour into glasses and enjoy immediately.

Nutritional Facts: (Per serving)

- ❖ **Calories:** 80
- ❖ **Vitamin C:** 120% of RDA
- ❖ **Anti-inflammatory agents:** High
- ❖ **Hydration:** Excellent

This Turmeric, Orange Ginger Smoothie is a refreshing and nutrient-dense drink that supports weight loss and provides a healthy dose of antioxidants. Enjoy this delicious smoothie for a morning pick-me-up or as a refreshing afternoon snack.

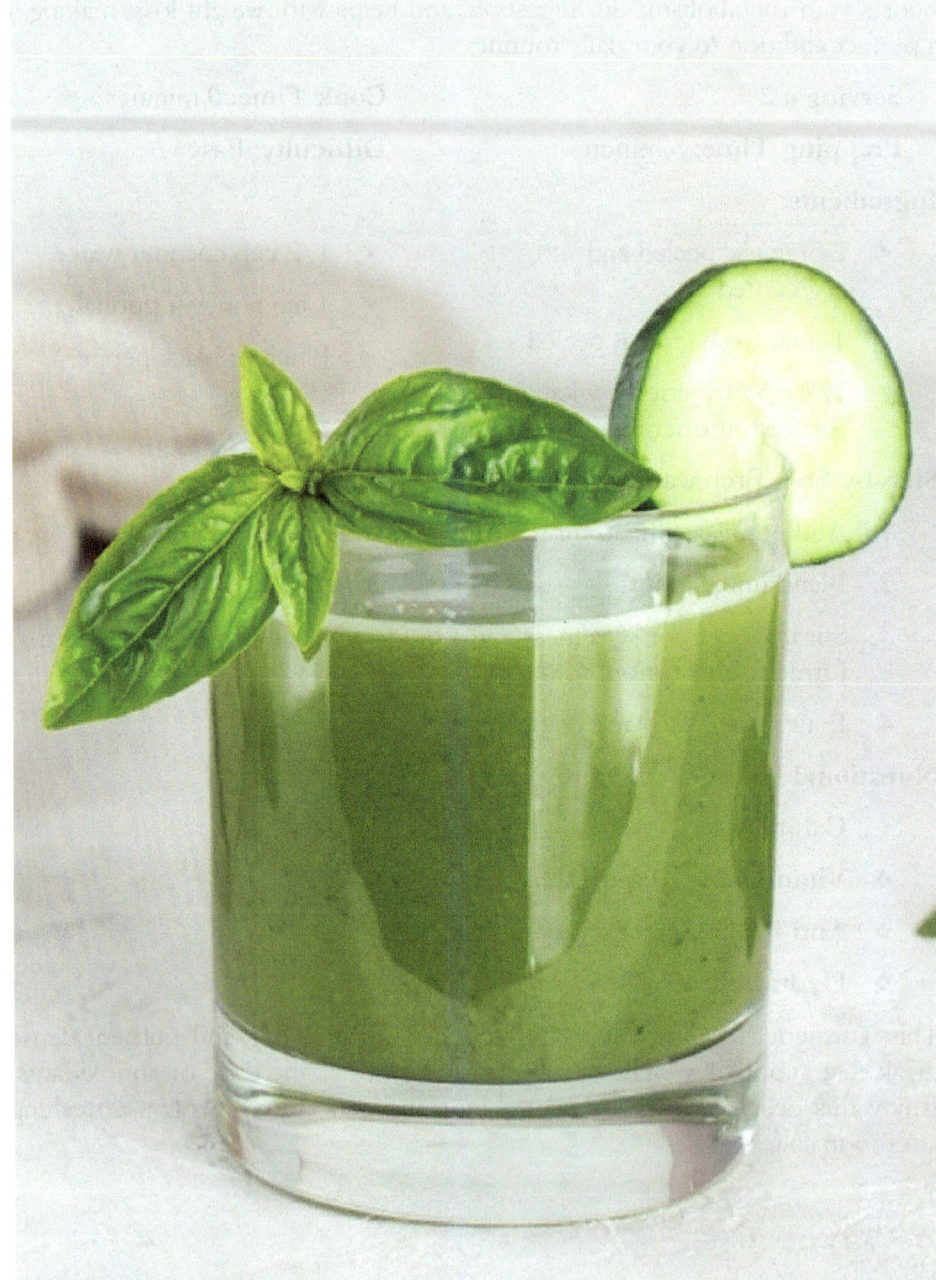

Cucumber Infused Detox Water

Cucumber-infused detox water is not just a refreshing and hydrating drink, it's a natural aid in weight loss. This drink helps flush out toxins, keeps you energized throughout the day, and supports your overall health and well-being.

Servings: 1

Prepping Time: 5 minutes

Cook Time: 0 minutes

Difficulty: Easy

Ingredients:

- ✓ 1 medium cucumber, thinly sliced
- ✓ 1 lemon, sliced
- ✓ 5-6 mint leaves
- ✓ 1-liter water
- ✓ Ice cubes (optional)

Step-by-Step Preparation:

1. Add cucumber, lemon slices, and mint leaves to a pitcher.
2. Pour water over the ingredients.
3. Let the mixture sit in the fridge for at least 1 hour.
4. Serve chilled with optional ice cubes.

Nutritional Facts (Per serving):

- ❖ **Calories**: 10
- ❖ **Carbohydrates**: 2g
- ❖ **Fat**: 0g
- ❖ **Protein**: 0g

By incorporating cucumber-infused detox water into your daily routine, you're taking a proactive step towards a healthier you. This easy-to-prepare, refreshing drink may support weight loss, keep you hydrated, and leave you feeling fresh all day, contributing to your overall well-being.

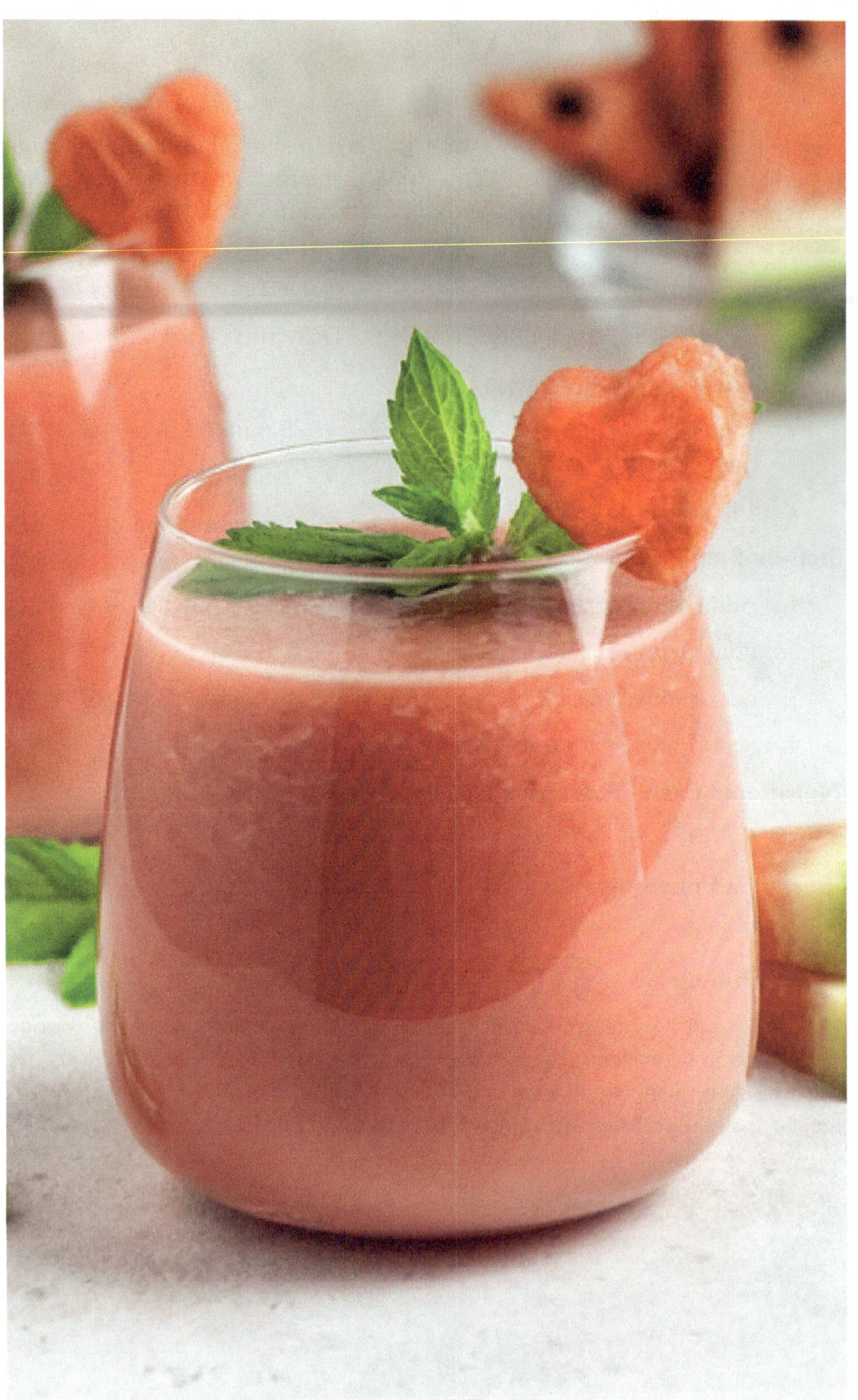

Watermelon Coconut Smoothie

Watermelon Coconut Smoothie is a light, hydrating, and tropical drink perfect for weight loss. The refreshing combination of watermelon and coconut not only satisfies your thirst but also helps boost your metabolism, keeps you full longer, and provides essential hydration, reassuring you of its health benefits.

Servings: 1

Prepping Time: 5 minutes

Cook Time: 0 minutes

Difficulty: Easy

Ingredients:

- ✓ 2 cups watermelon, cubed
- ✓ 1/2 cup coconut water
- ✓ 1 tablespoon lime juice
- ✓ 1 teaspoon chia seeds
- ✓ Ice cubes (optional)

Step-by-Step Preparation:

1. Add watermelon, coconut water, and lime juice to a blender.
2. Blend until smooth.
3. Stir in chia seeds.
4. Pour into a glass and serve chilled with optional ice cubes.

Nutritional Facts (Per serving):

- ❖ **Calories**: 60
- ❖ **Carbohydrates**: 15g
- ❖ **Fat**: 1g
- ❖ **Protein**: 1g

This Watermelon Coconut Smoothie is not just a one-time treat, but a versatile companion for your weight loss journey. Whether you enjoy it as a post-workout refresher, a mid-morning pick-me-up, or a satisfying dessert, this smoothie is always a delicious and healthy choice.

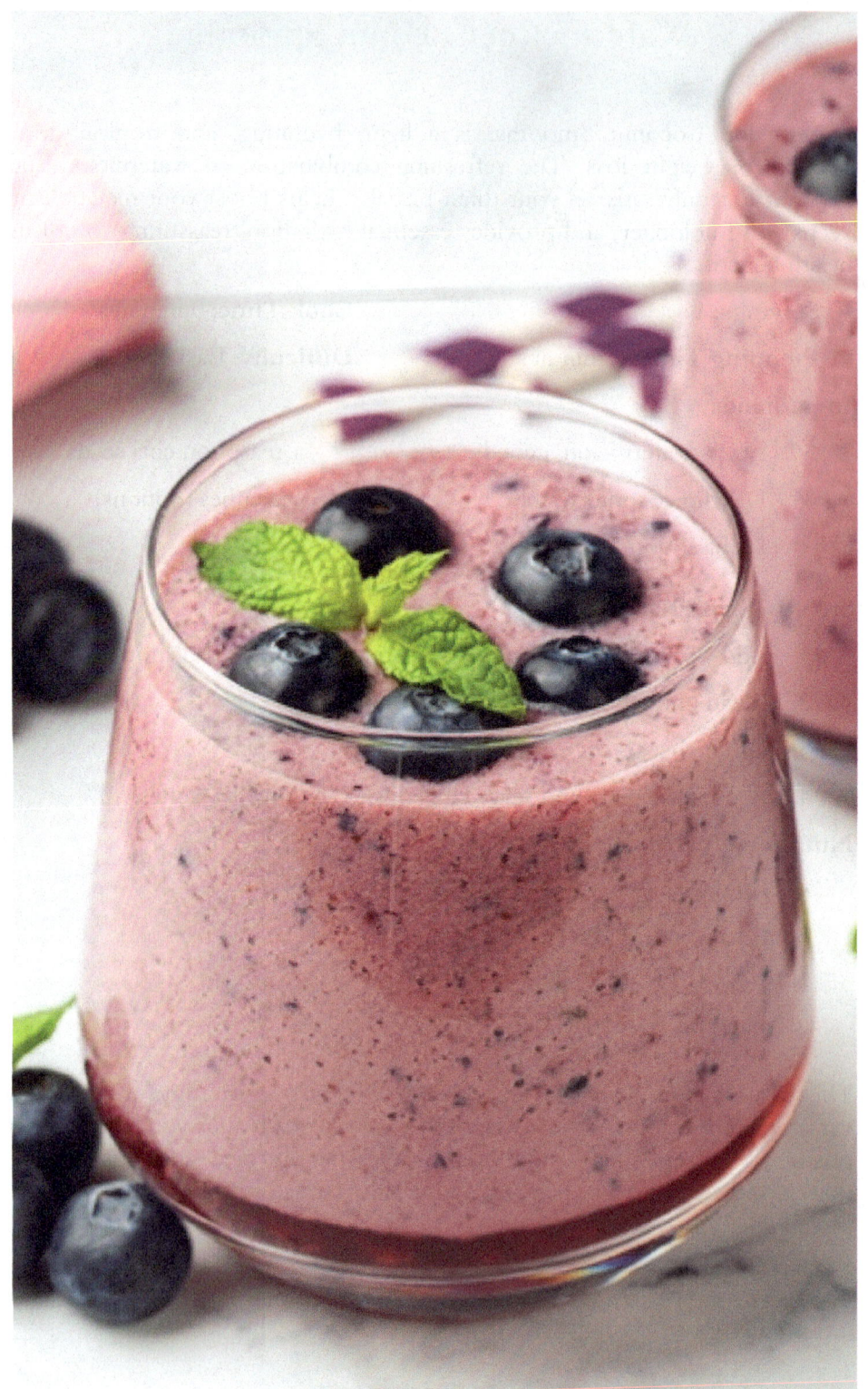

Fruit-Based Juices

Blueberry Smoothie With Mint and Fresh Berries

The Blueberry Smoothie with Mint and Fresh Berries is not just a refreshing, antioxidant-packed drink. It is also a supportive companion in your weight loss journey. The tangy berries and cooling mint blend together to offer a burst of revitalizing flavor, while the low-calorie, high-nutrient content keeps you full and satisfied, reassuring you of its health benefits.

Servings: 1

Prepping Time: 5 minutes

Cook Time: 0 minutes

Difficulty: Easy

Ingredients:

- ✓ 1/2 cup fresh blueberries
- ✓ 1/4 cup mixed fresh berries (strawberries, raspberries)
- ✓ 1 tablespoon fresh mint leaves
- ✓ 1/2 cup unsweetened almond milk
- ✓ 1 teaspoon chia seeds
- ✓ Ice cubes (optional)

Step-by-Step Preparation:

1. Add blueberries, mixed berries, mint, and almond milk to a blender.
2. Blend until smooth.
3. Stir in chia seeds.
4. Serve chilled, with ice cubes if desired.

Nutritional Facts (Per serving):

- ❖ **Calories**: 80
- ❖ **Carbohydrates**: 15g
- ❖ **Fat**: 2g
- ❖ **Protein**: 2g

This Blueberry Smoothie with Mint and Fresh Berries is a delightful, low-calorie beverage that helps you stay energized and hydrated. Perfect for a quick breakfast or post-workout refreshment, it fits seamlessly into a balanced, weight-conscious lifestyle. It's best consumed immediately, but can be stored in the refrigerator for up to 24 hours.

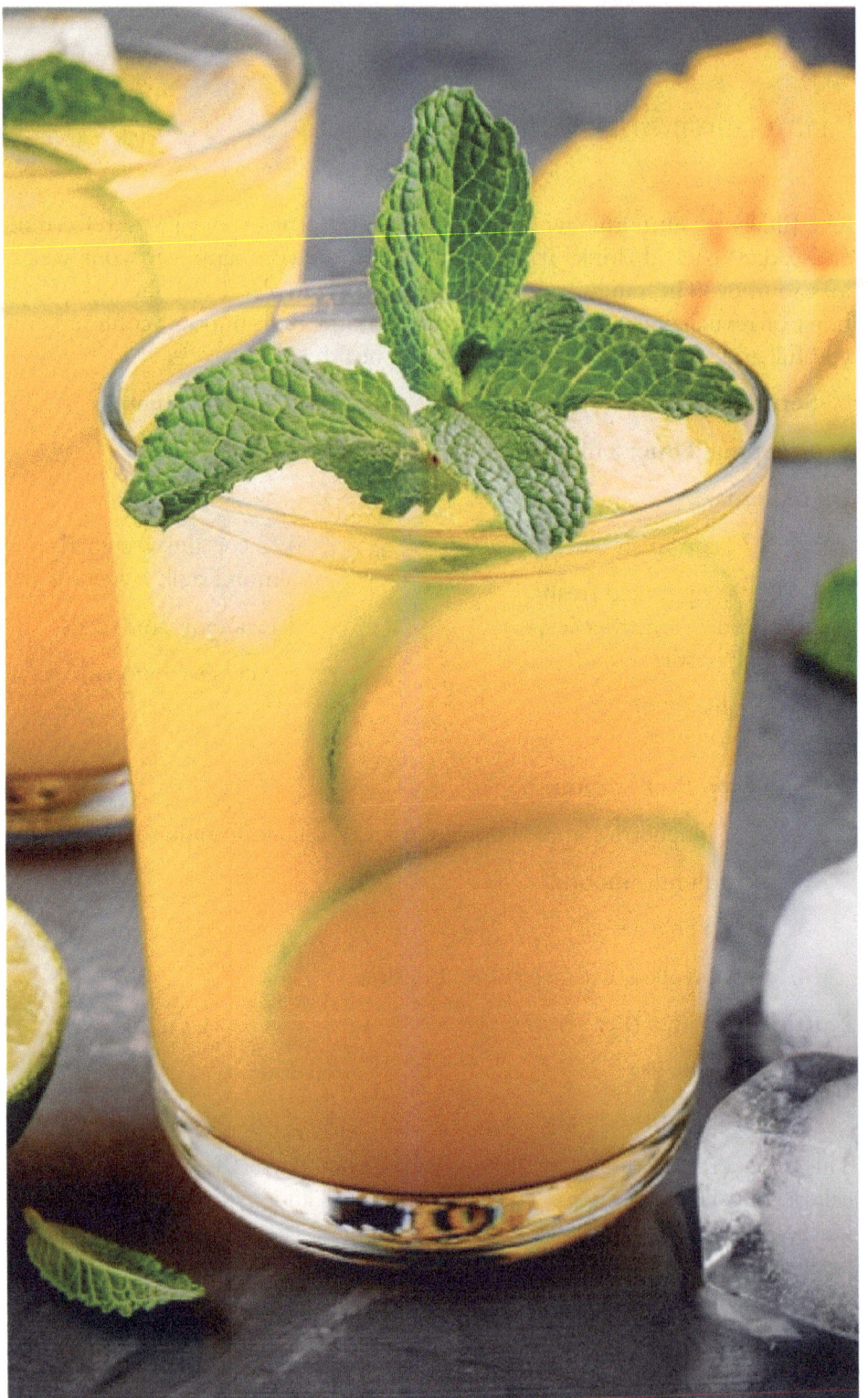

Mango Lemonade With Lime and Mint

Mango Lemonade with Lime and Mint is a refreshing, tangy drink perfect for weight loss. The combination of mango, lemon, and lime provides a vitamin-rich boost, while mint adds a cooling touch. This hydrating juice not only helps curb cravings and aids digestion but also supports your weight loss goals, making it a great addition to your daily routine.

Servings: 1

Cook Time: 0 minutes

Prepping Time: 5 minutes

Difficulty: Easy

Ingredients:

- ✓ 1/2 cup ripe mango, cubed
- ✓ Juice of 1 lemon
- ✓ Juice of 1/2 lime
- ✓ 5-6 fresh mint leaves
- ✓ 1 cup cold water
- ✓ Ice cubes (optional)

Step-by-Step Preparation:

1. Blend mango, lemon juice, lime juice, and water until smooth.
2. Add mint leaves and pulse briefly.
3. Serve chilled with ice cubes, if desired.

Nutritional Facts (Per serving):

- ❖ **Calories**: 70
- ❖ **Carbohydrates**: 18g
- ❖ **Fat**: 0g
- ❖ **Protein**: 1g

This Mango Lemonade with Lime and Mint is a refreshing way to stay hydrated and support your weight loss goals. Easy to prepare, it's a delightful drink to enjoy anytime. Feel free to experiment with different fruits and herbs to create your own unique variations, all while helping you feel revitalized and refreshed.

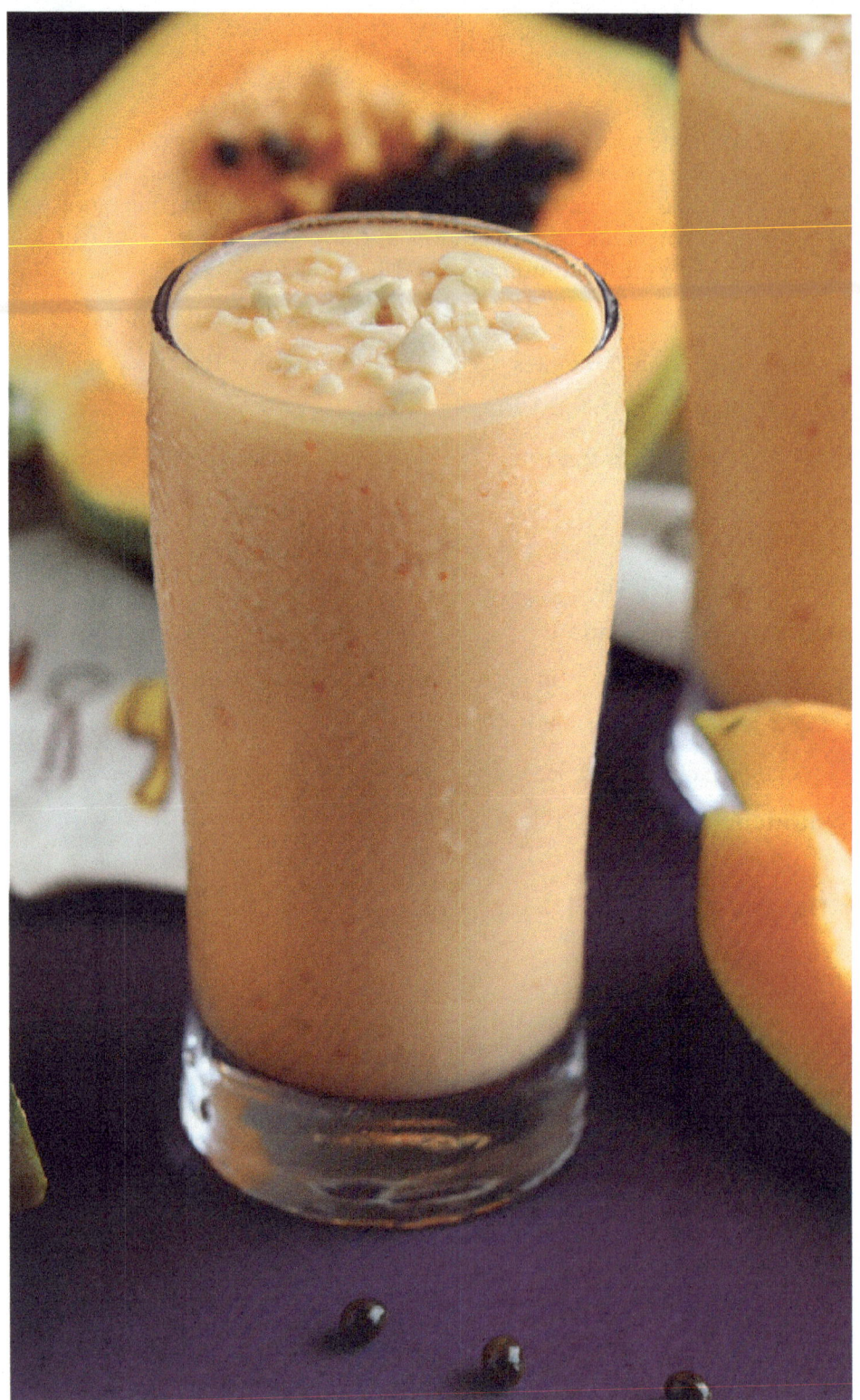

Papaya Milk Shake

Papaya Milkshake is not just a delicious treat, but also a health booster. Made with ripe papaya, milk, and a scoop of vanilla ice cream, this creamy drink is rich in vitamins and fiber. It aids digestion and supports weight loss, making it a smart choice for those conscious about their health. The natural sweetness of papaya and the creamy texture create a perfect balance for a satisfying yet healthy treat.

Servings: 1

Prepping Time: 5 minutes

Cook Time: 0 minutes

Difficulty: Easy

Ingredients:

- ✓ 1 cup ripe papaya, cubed
- ✓ 1/2 cup low-fat milk
- ✓ 1 scoop vanilla ice cream
- ✓ Ice cubes (optional)

Step-by-Step Preparation:

1. Add papaya, milk, and ice cream to a blender.
2. Blend until smooth and creamy.
3. Serve chilled, with optional ice cubes.

Nutritional Facts (Per serving):

- ❖ **Calories**: 150
- ❖ **Carbohydrates**: 25g
- ❖ **Fat**: 4g
- ❖ **Protein**: 4g

With its refreshing taste and fiber-rich goodness, this Papaya Milkshake is a perfect choice for those looking to lose weight without sacrificing flavor. Its smooth texture and tropical taste make it a delightful breakfast or afternoon snack choice. Moreover, the best part? It is so easy to make, you can enjoy the natural goodness of papaya while staying on track with your goals!

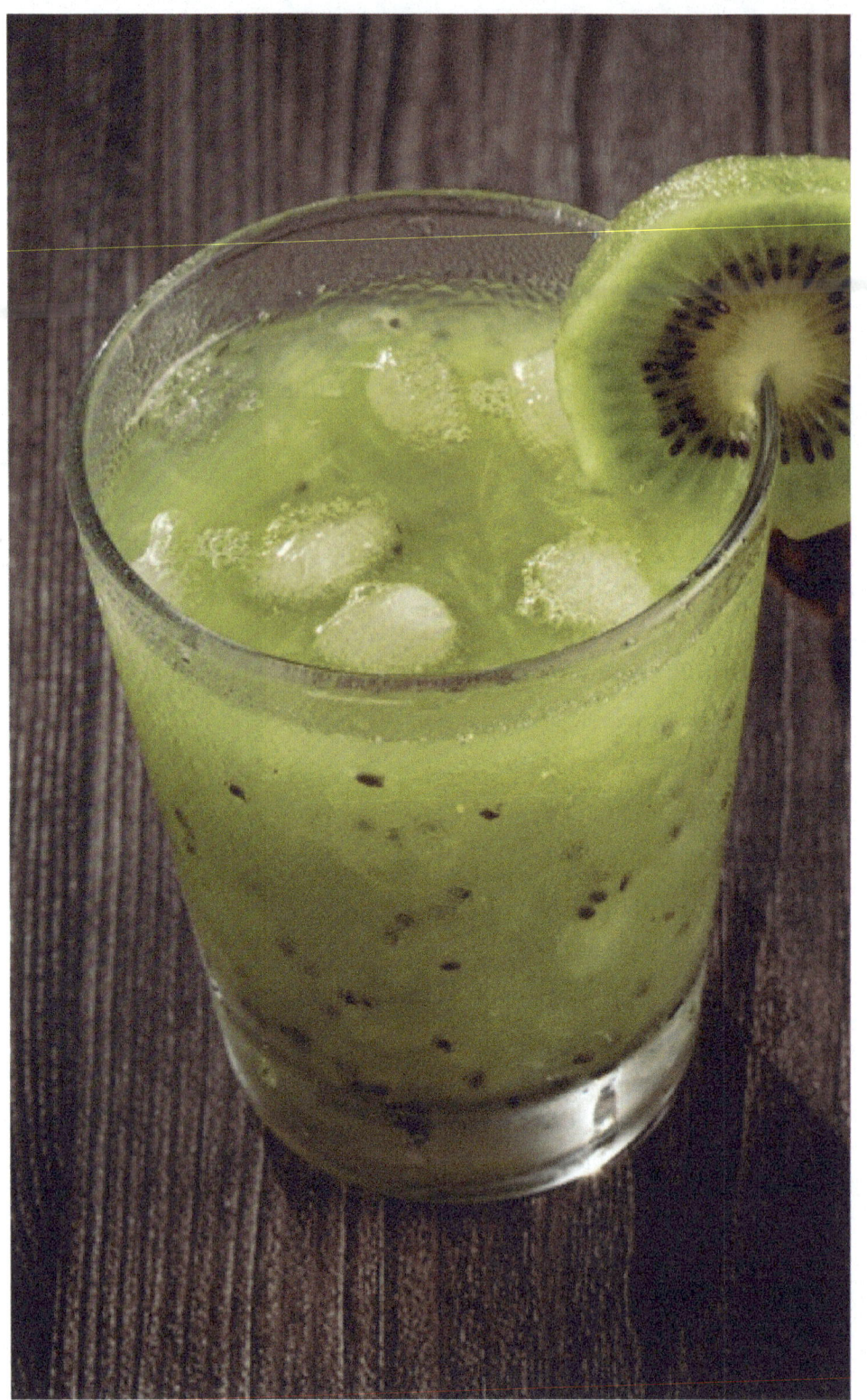

Kiwi Caipirinha

The Kiwi Caipirinha is not just a delicious beverage, it is a health booster. This zesty, tropical drink combines the tangy flavor of fresh kiwi with lime, creating a refreshing, low-calorie juice that is packed with vitamins and antioxidants. It is a perfect choice for those looking to hydrate and boost their daily metabolism, knowing they are also getting a nutrient-rich drink.

Servings: 1

Prepping Time: 5 minutes

Cook Time: 0 minutes

Difficulty: Easy

Ingredients:

- ✓ 2 ripe kiwis, peeled and diced
- ✓ Juice of 1 lime
- ✓ 1 teaspoon honey or sweetener of choice
- ✓ 1/2 cup cold water
- ✓ Ice cubes (optional)

Step-by-Step Preparation:

1. Add diced kiwi and lime juice to a blender.
2. Blend until smooth.
3. Stir in honey and cold water.
4. Serve chilled with ice cubes if desired.

Nutritional Facts (Per serving):

- ❖ **Calories**: 70
- ❖ **Carbohydrates**: 18g
- ❖ **Fat**: 0g
- ❖ **Protein**: 1g

The Kiwi Caipirinha is not just a weight loss support, it's a versatile drink that can accompany you throughout the day. Whether you need a refreshing start to your morning, a midday pick-me-up, or a relaxing evening beverage, this revitalizing, tangy drink is there for you. It is easy to prepare, nutrient-rich, and a flavorful way to nourish your body and support your health goals.

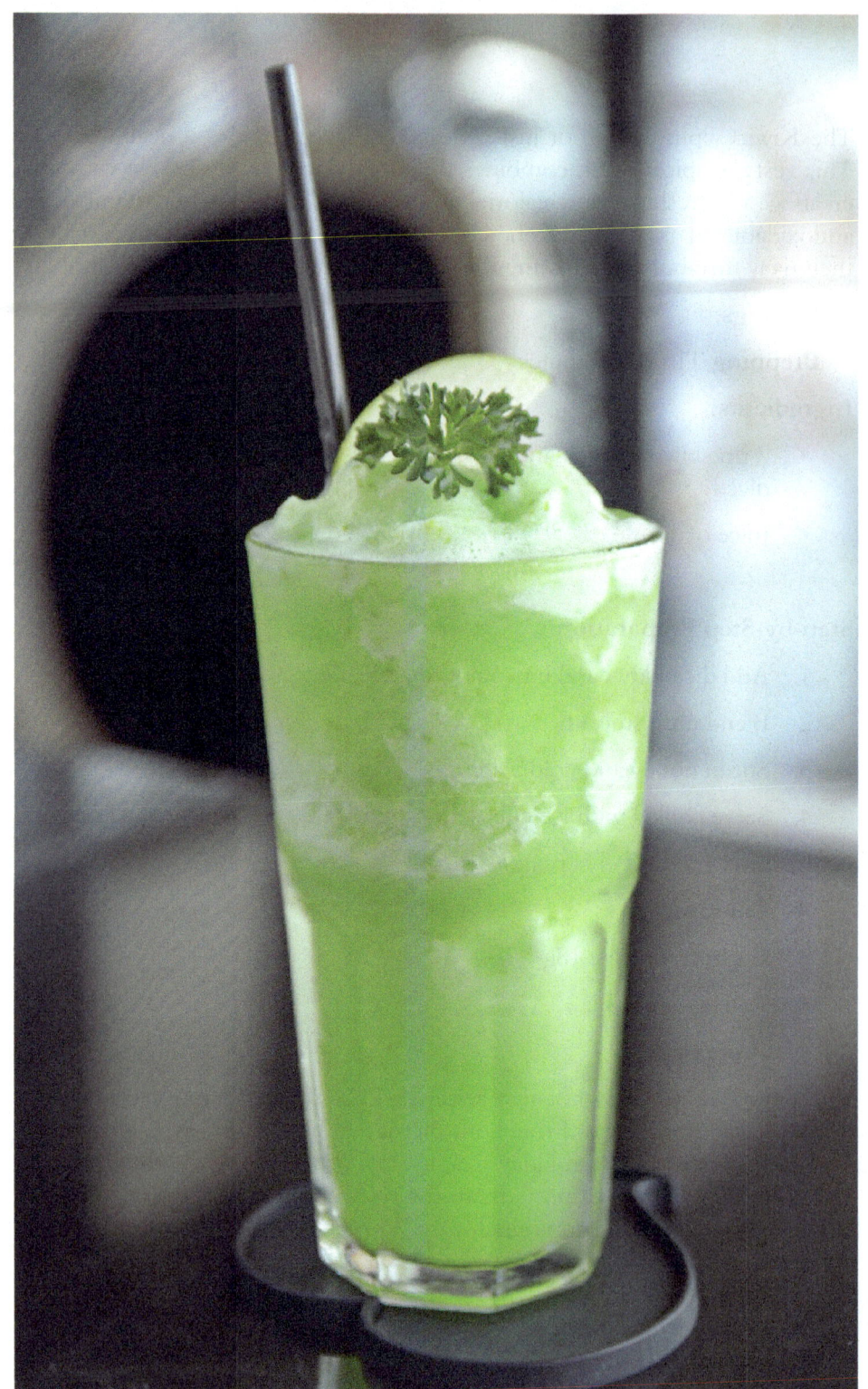

Green Apple Smoothie

Green Apple Smoothie is a refreshing and nutritious drink for weight loss. The tartness of green apples, combined with the fiber and vitamins, makes this smoothie an excellent metabolism booster. It is light and hydrating and keeps you feeling full, helping curb cravings throughout the day.

Servings: 1

Prepping Time: 5 minutes

Cook Time: 0 minutes

Difficulty: Easy

Ingredients:

- ✓ 1 medium green apple, chopped
- ✓ 1/2 cup spinach leaves
- ✓ 1/2 cup unsweetened almond milk
- ✓ 1 tablespoon chia seeds
- ✓ 1 teaspoon lemon juice
- ✓ Ice cubes (optional)

Step-by-Step Preparation:

1. Add green apple, spinach, almond milk, and lemon juice to a blender.
2. Blend until smooth.
3. Stir in chia seeds.
4. Serve chilled with optional ice cubes.

Nutritional Facts (Per serving):

- ❖ **Calories**: 90
- ❖ **Carbohydrates**: 20g
- ❖ **Fat**: 2g
- ❖ **Protein**: 2g

This Green Apple Smoothie is a delicious way to start your day or enjoy as a mid-morning or afternoon snack. Its rich fiber content helps with digestion and weight loss while keeping you energized and satisfied. It is a simple, healthy, and tasty choice for your daily routine.

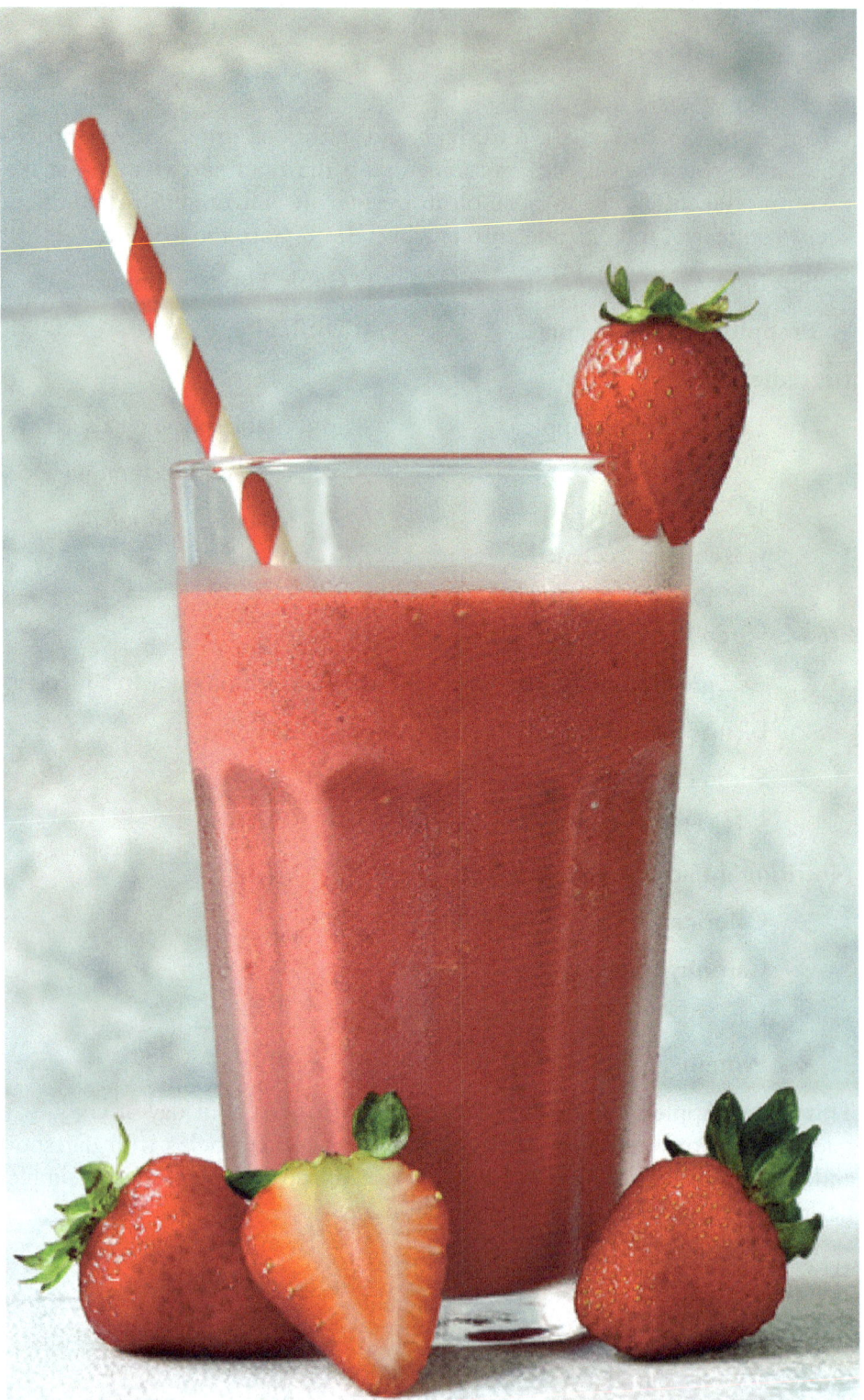

Strawberry Milkshake

Strawberry Milkshake is not just a delicious treat, but also a powerhouse of health benefits. Packed with antioxidants, vitamins, and fiber, this creamy drink not only satisfies your cravings but also supports your health goals. With just a few ingredients, it is easy to whip up and enjoy any time of the day.

Servings: 1

Cook Time: 2 minutes

Prepping Time: 5 minutes

Difficulty: Easy

Ingredients:

- ✓ 1 cup fresh strawberries
- ✓ 1 cup almond milk (unsweetened)
- ✓ 1 tbsp chia seeds
- ✓ 1 tsp honey (optional)
- ✓ Ice cubes (optional)

Step-by-Step Preparation:

1. Wash and hull the strawberries.
2. Blend strawberries, almond milk, chia seeds, and honey until smooth.
3. Add ice cubes for a chilled texture if desired.
4. Serve immediately.

Nutritional Facts (Per serving):

- ❖ **Calories:** 120
- ❖ **Sugar:** 10g
- ❖ **Protein:** 3g
- ❖ **Fat:** 3g
- ❖ **Fiber:** 5g

Enjoy this strawberry milkshake as a guilt-free, delicious way to fuel your body. Whether as a snack or meal replacement, it helps promote healthy digestion and boosts energy. You can also experiment with different toppings or add-ins to create your own unique version, making it an ideal choice for weight loss goals.

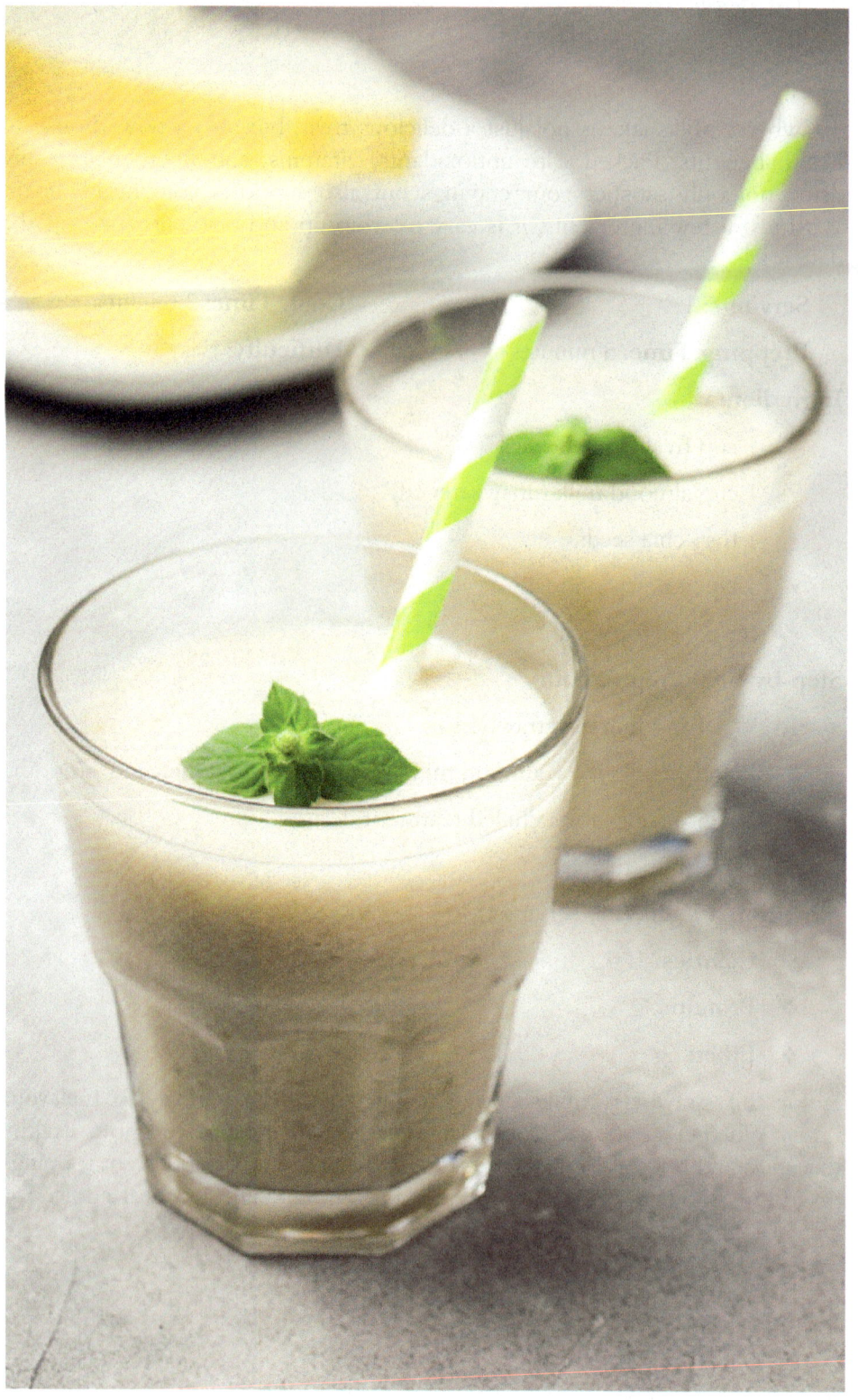

Cantaloupe Melon Mint

The Cantaloupe Melon Mint Smoothie is not just a refreshing and hydrating drink, it's a powerhouse of health benefits. This low-calorie, nutrient-rich drink is packed with vitamins, antioxidants, and fiber. With a hint of mint, it offers a cooling and revitalizing boost, making it a great addition to your healthy diet plan.

Servings: 2

Prepping Time: 5 minutes

Cook Time: 2 minutes

Difficulty: Easy

Ingredients:

- ✓ 2 cups cantaloupe melon (cubed)
- ✓ 1/2 cup coconut water
- ✓ 5-6 fresh mint leaves
- ✓ 1 tsp lime juice
- ✓ Ice cubes (optional)

Step-by-Step Preparation:

1. Add cantaloupe melon cubes, coconut water, mint leaves, and lime juice to a blender.
2. Blend until smooth and creamy.
3. Add ice cubes for a chilled texture if desired.
4. Serve immediately and enjoy.

Nutritional Facts (Per serving):

- ❖ **Calories:** 90
- ❖ **Protein:** 1g
- ❖ **Fiber:** 2g
- ❖ **Sugar:** 18g
- ❖ **Fat:** 0g

This cantaloupe melon mint smoothie is a delicious and light option to help you stay full and hydrated while supporting your weight loss goals. It's refreshing taste makes it a perfect snack or post-workout drink.

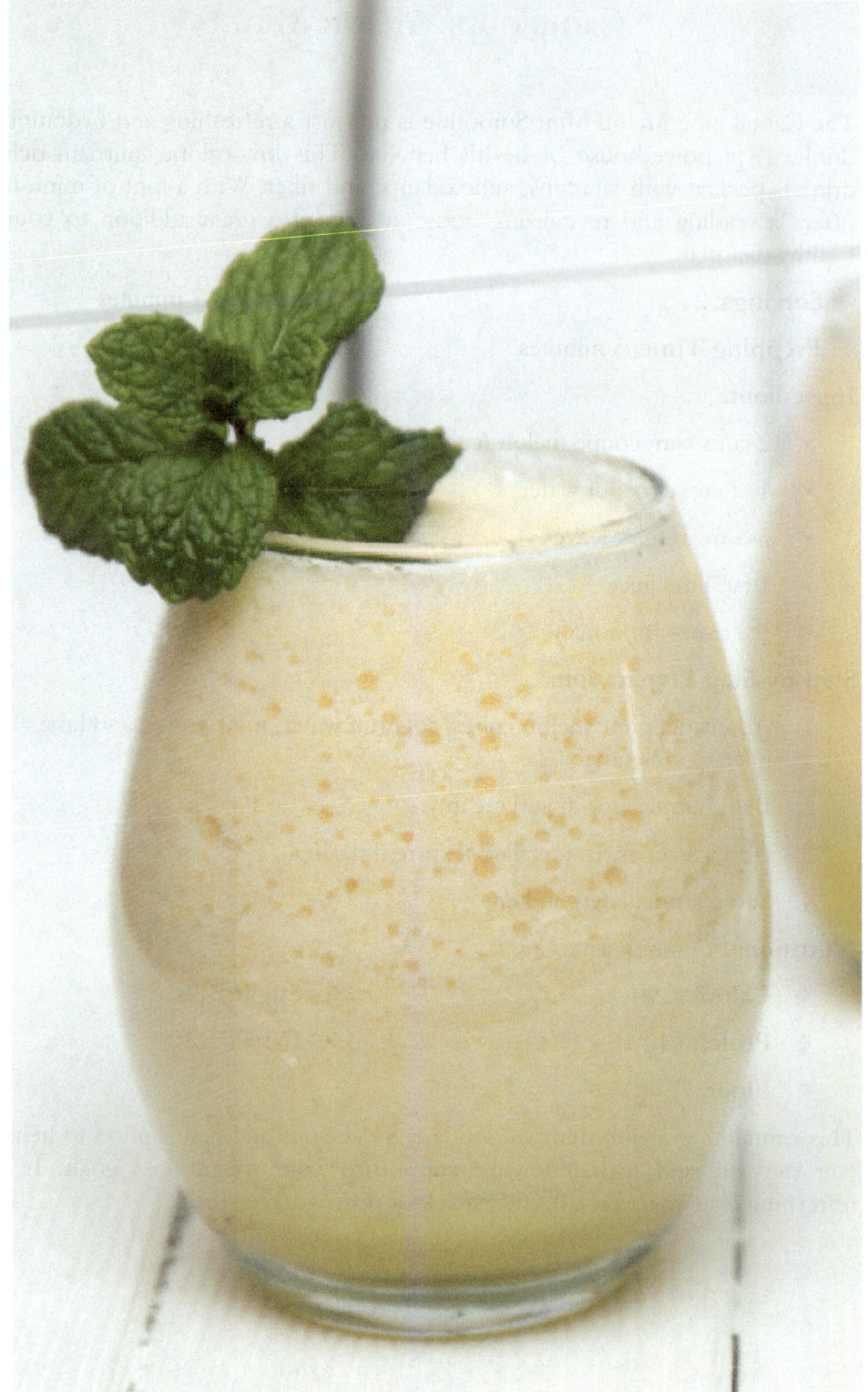

Fresh Pineapple Juice is a naturally sweet and tangy drink, perfect for weight loss. Loaded with digestive enzymes and antioxidants, it helps reduce bloating and boosts metabolism. This simple, refreshing juice is a great way to stay hydrated and support your health goals with minimal calories.

Servings: 1

Cook Time: 2 minutes

Prepping Time: 5 minutes

Difficulty: Easy

Ingredients:

- ✓ 1 cup fresh pineapple (cubed)
- ✓ 1/2 cup cold water
- ✓ 1 tsp lemon juice
- ✓ Ice cubes (optional)

Step-by-Step Preparation:

1. Add pineapple cubes, cold water, and lemon juice to a blender.
2. Blend until smooth.
3. Strain the juice if you prefer a smoother texture.
4. Serve with ice cubes if desired.

Nutritional Facts (Per serving):

- ❖ **Calories:** 100
- ❖ **Protein:** 1g
- ❖ **Fiber:** 2g
- ❖ **Sugar:** 19g
- ❖ **Fat:** 0g

Enjoy this fresh pineapple juice as a hydrating, vitamin-rich option to keep you full and energized. It is a perfect addition to a weight loss routine, helping to curb cravings while offering essential nutrients. For best results, consume it in the morning or as a mid-day snack.

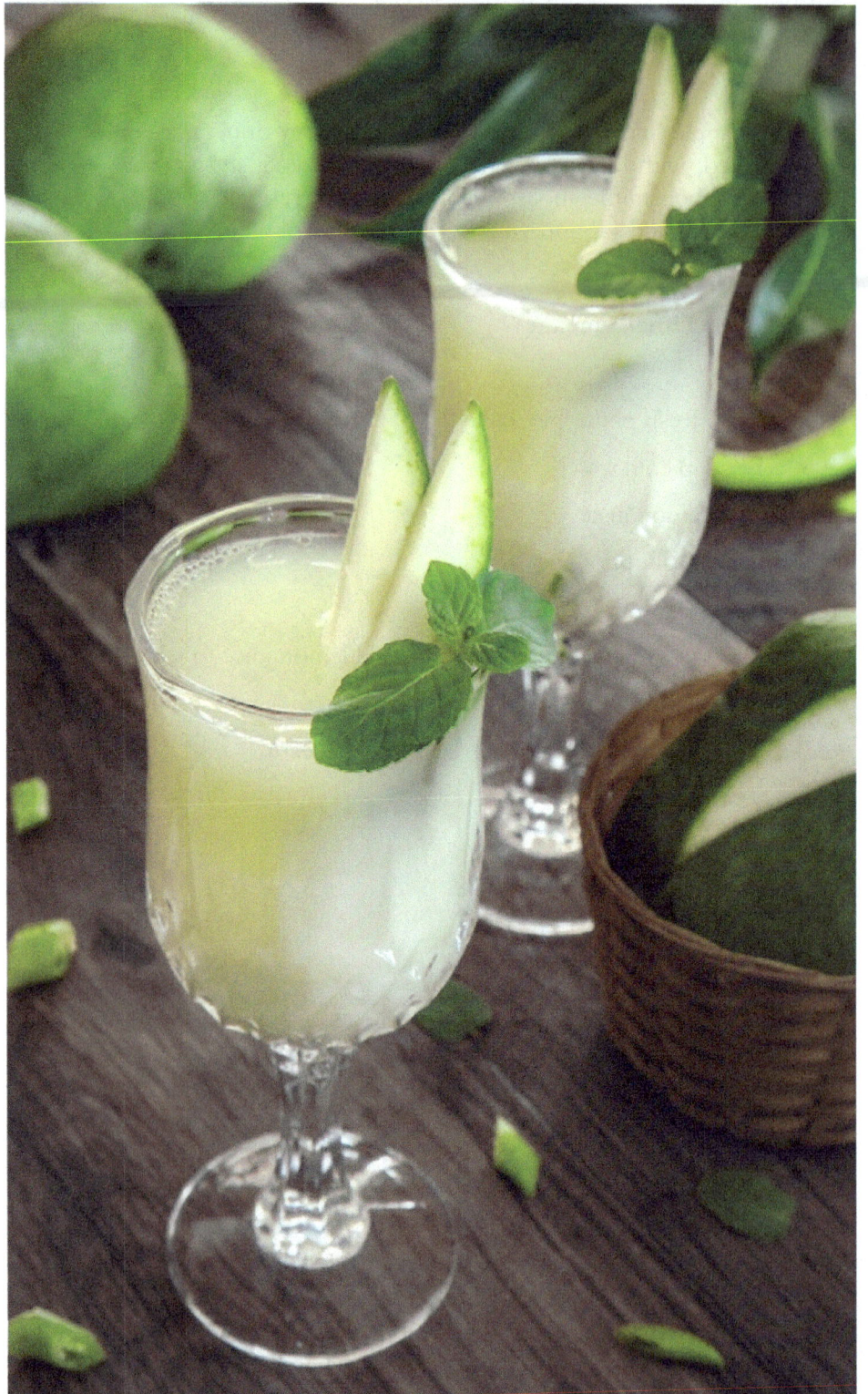

Raw Mango Juice is not just a delicious and refreshing drink, but also a powerhouse of essential vitamins and minerals. Packed with the goodness of raw mangoes, this hydrating juice is a perfect companion for your weight-loss journey. It aids digestion, curbs cravings, and boosts metabolism, all while keeping your calorie intake in check. It is a great choice for a healthy summer detox.

Servings: 2

Cook Time: 0 minutes

Prepping Time: 10 minutes

Difficulty: Easy

Ingredients:

- ✓ 2 raw mangoes, peeled and chopped
- ✓ 2 cups water
- ✓ 1 tablespoon honey (optional)
- ✓ A pinch of black salt
- ✓ A few mint leaves for garnish
- ✓ Ice cubes (optional)

Step-by-Step Preparation:

1. Blend the raw mango pieces with water until smooth.
2. Strain the mixture to remove any pulp.
3. Add honey and black salt and mix well.
4. Pour the juice into glasses, add ice cubes, and garnish with mint leaves.
5. Serve chilled.

Nutritional Facts (Per serving):

- ❖ **Calories**: 80
- ❖ **Protein**: 1g
- ❖ **Fiber**: 2g
- ❖ **Carbs**: 22g
- ❖ **Fat**: 0g

This raw mango juice is not just a delicious beverage, it's a powerhouse of health benefits. With just 80 calories per serving, it is a low-calorie option that keeps you full and energized throughout the day. Packed with vitamins A and C, it is a perfect refreshing drink to support your weight-loss goals while enhancing digestion and hydration.

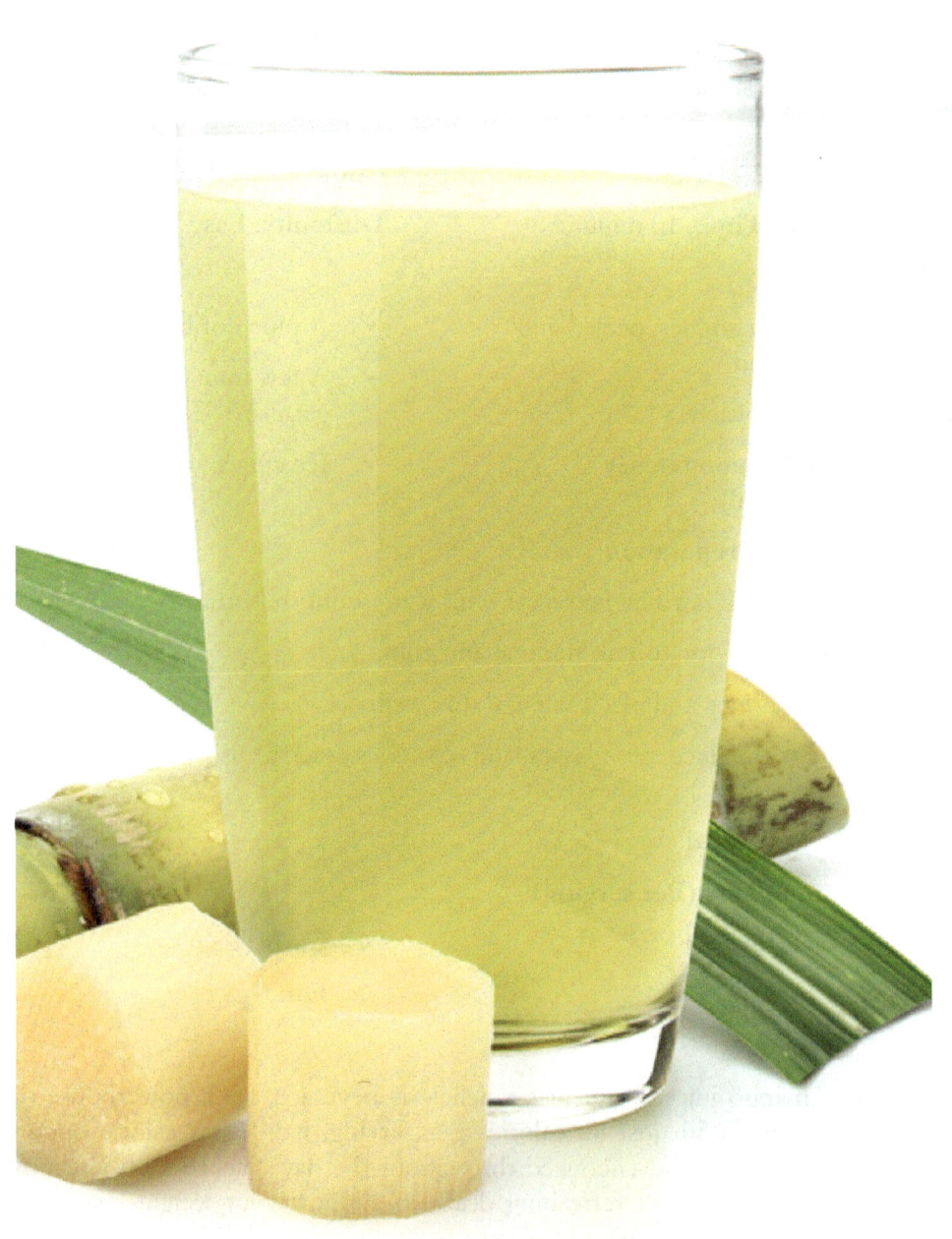

Squeezed Sugar Cane Juice

Sugar cane juice, a natural and refreshing drink, is not just a treat for your taste buds, but also a boon for your health. It aids in weight loss, is rich in essential nutrients, and is a powerhouse of antioxidants. With its low fat content, it is a perfect fit for your balanced diet. This simple and hydrating juice can boost your metabolism and keep you feeling full longer, ensuring you stay healthy and fit.

Servings: 1

Prepping Time: 5 minutes

Cook Time: 0 minutes

Difficulty: Easy

Ingredients:

- ✓ 1 large sugar cane stalk, peeled and cut into pieces
- ✓ 1/2 lemon (optional)
- ✓ A pinch of black salt (optional)
- ✓ Ice cubes (optional)

Step-by-Step Preparation:

1. Place sugar cane pieces in a juicer.
2. Collect the fresh juice and strain if needed.
3. Squeeze in lemon juice and add black salt for flavor, if desired.
4. Serve over ice for a chilled experience.

Nutritional Facts (Per serving):

- ❖ **Calories:** 130
- ❖ **Protein:** 0g
- ❖ **Fiber:** 0g
- ❖ **Carbs:** 34g
- ❖ **Fat:** 0g

Enjoy this hydrating sugar cane juice as part of your weight loss routine. Its low in calories, provides natural energy, and supports digestion, making it the perfect refreshing beverage to keep you on track. However, if you have diabetes or are watching your sugar intake, it is best to consume this juice in moderation.

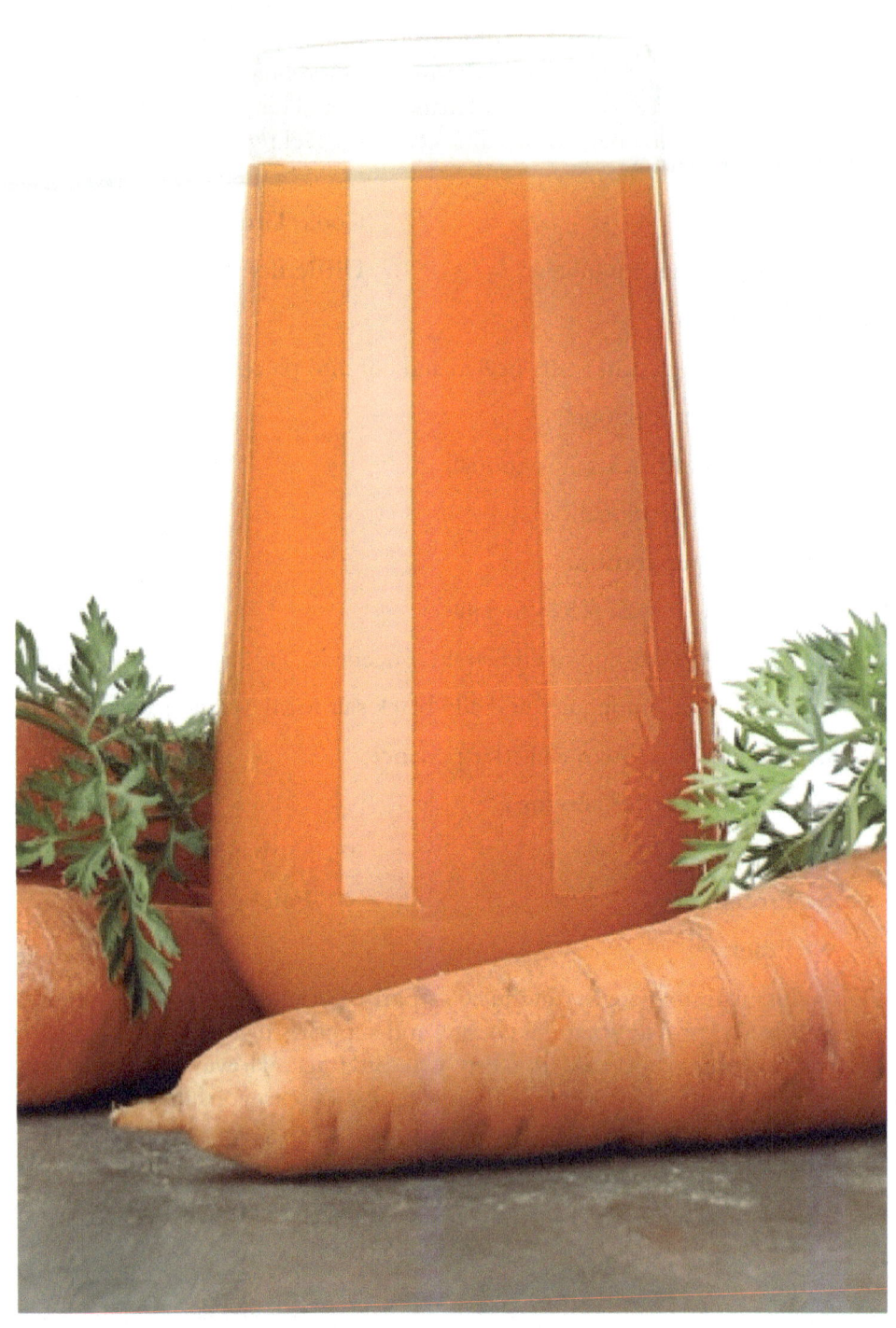

Plant-Based Juices

Carrot Ginger Delight

Carrot Ginger Juice is a vibrant and nutrient-packed drink ideal for weight loss. Rich in antioxidants, vitamins, and anti-inflammatory properties, it boosts metabolism and helps detoxify the body. With the natural sweetness of carrots and the zing of ginger, it is a refreshing way to stay hydrated while supporting your health goals.

Servings: 1

Prepping Time: 5 minutes

Cook Time: 0 minutes

Difficulty: Easy

Ingredients:

- ✓ 3 medium carrots, peeled and chopped
- ✓ 1-inch piece of fresh ginger, peeled
- ✓ 1/2 lemon, juiced
- ✓ 1/2 cup water
- ✓ Ice cubes (optional)

Step-by-Step Preparation:

1. Place the chopped carrots and ginger into a juicer.
2. Add water and blend until smooth.
3. Strain the juice and discard any pulp.
4. Stir in lemon juice and mix well.
5. Serve over ice if desired.

Nutritional Facts (Per serving):

- ❖ **Calories:** 90
- ❖ **Protein:** 1g
- ❖ **Fiber:** 3g
- ❖ **Carbs:** 22g
- ❖ **Fat:** 0g

Carrot Ginger Juice is not just a delicious drink, it's a powerhouse of health benefits. This wholesome, low-calorie drink provides a natural energy boost, aids digestion, and supports weight loss. Packed with vitamin A and antioxidants, it is a perfect choice for those looking to stay refreshed and light throughout the day. Knowing that each sip is contributing to your health and wellness can be a great source of motivation and inspiration.

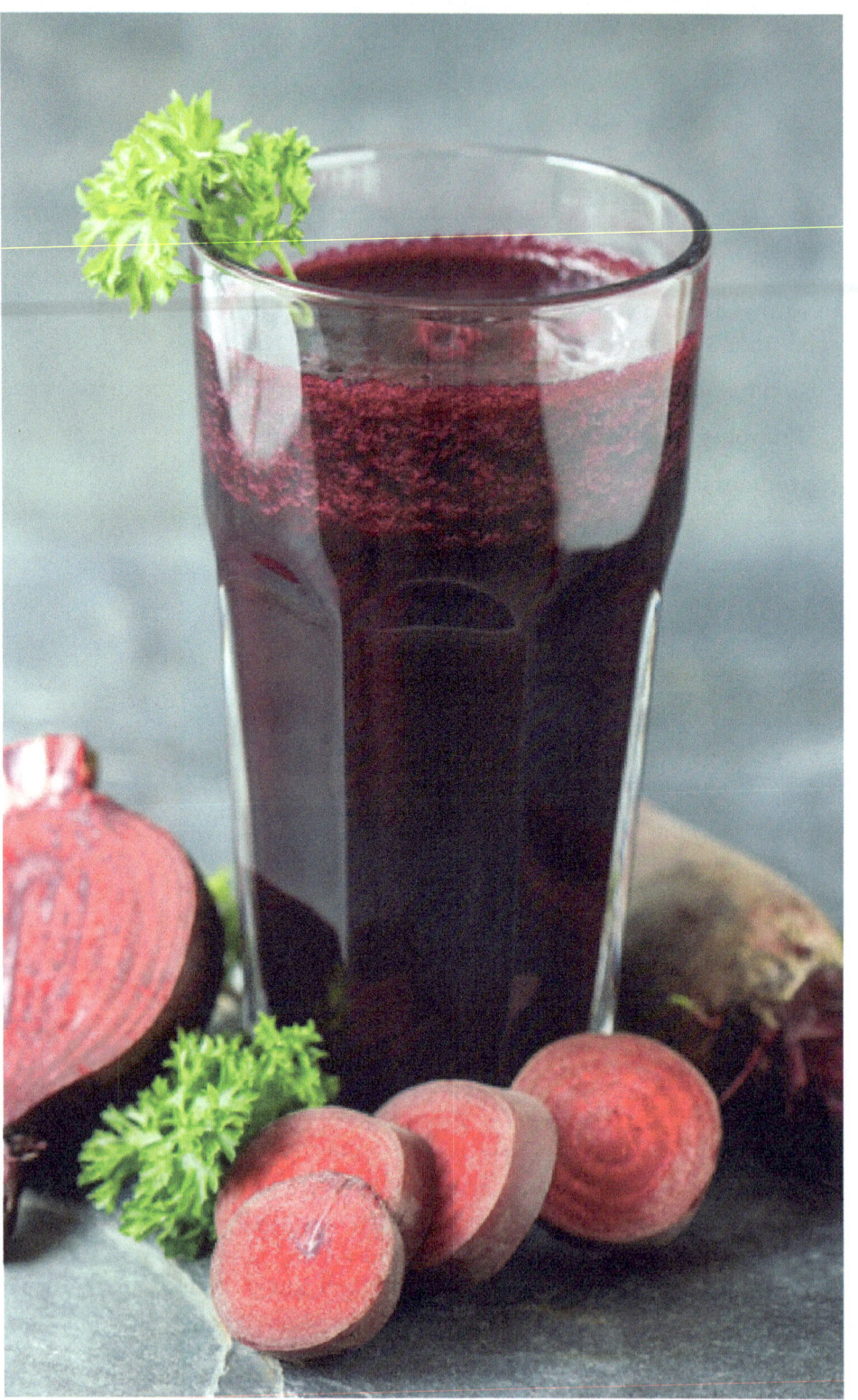

Beet Powerhouse Juice

Healthy Beetroot Juice is a powerhouse of nutrients, making it a perfect choice for weight loss. Loaded with fiber, antioxidants, and essential vitamins, this juice helps detoxify the body, boost stamina, and improve digestion. Its natural sweetness and earthy flavor make it a refreshing and satisfying drink that keeps your energy up while cutting calories.

Servings: 1

Prepping Time: 10 minutes

Cook Time: 0 minutes

Difficulty: Easy

Ingredients:

- ✓ 1 medium beetroot, peeled and chopped
- ✓ 1 small apple, chopped
- ✓ 1-inch piece of ginger, peeled
- ✓ 1/2 lemon, juiced
- ✓ 1/2 cup water
- ✓ Ice cubes (optional)

Step-by-Step Preparation:

1. Add beetroot, apple, and ginger to a blender.
2. Add water and blend until smooth.
3. Strain the juice to remove the pulp.
4. Stir in lemon juice and mix well.
5. Serve over ice if preferred.

Nutritional Facts (Per serving):

- ❖ **Calories**: 100
- ❖ **Protein**: 1g
- ❖ **Fiber**: 3g
- ❖ **Carbs**: 24g
- ❖ **Fat**: 0g

Healthy Beetroot Juice is not just a delicious drink, it's a powerhouse of health benefits. With its low-calorie, nutrient-dense composition, it is a great support for your weight loss journey. Packed with vitamins and minerals, it is a natural energy and metabolism booster, making it a perfect addition to your daily routine for a healthier you.

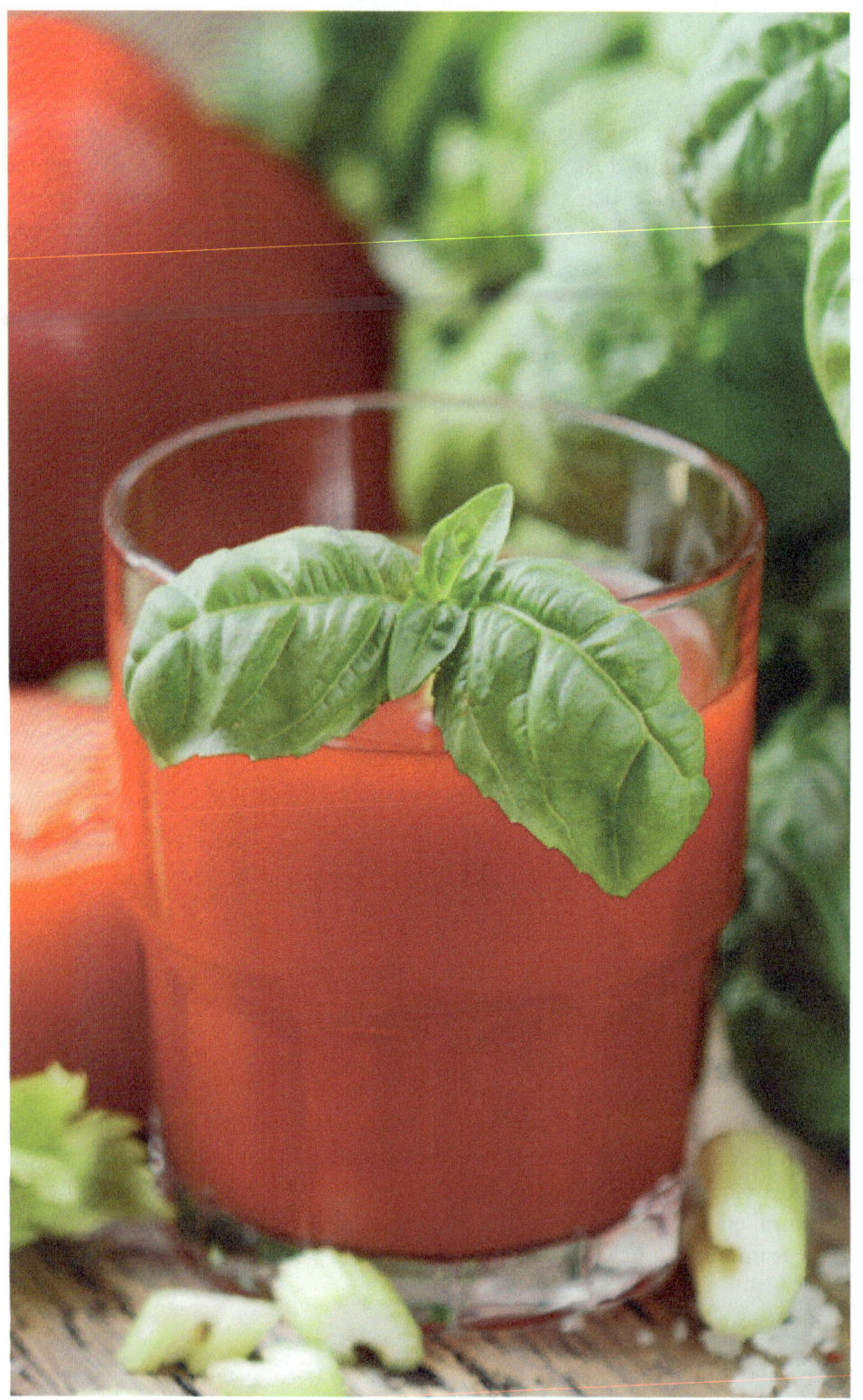

Tomato Basil Refresher

This Vegetable Juice from tomatoes, celery, and basil is a refreshing, low-calorie drink that supports weight loss. Rich in vitamins, minerals, and antioxidants, it helps cleanse your body while keeping you full and hydrated. The combination of tangy tomatoes, crunchy celery, and aromatic basil makes this juice a delicious and nutritious choice for any time of day.

Servings: 1

Prepping Time: 5 minutes

Cook Time: 0 minutes

Difficulty: Easy

Ingredients:

- ✓ 2 medium tomatoes, chopped
- ✓ 2 celery stalks, chopped
- ✓ A handful of fresh basil leaves
- ✓ 1/2 cup water
- ✓ A pinch of salt and pepper
- ✓ Ice cubes (optional)

Step-by-Step Preparation:

1. Blend tomatoes, celery, and basil with water until smooth.
2. Strain the juice to remove the pulp if preferred.
3. Add salt and pepper to taste, and stir well.
4. Pour over ice if desired and serve immediately.

Nutritional Facts (Per serving):

- ❖ **Calories**: 50
- ❖ **Protein**: 2g
- ❖ **Fiber**: 3g
- ❖ **Carbs**: 11g
- ❖ **Fat**: 0g

This vegetable juice is not just a delicious drink, but also a powerhouse of health benefits. It aids digestion, detoxifies the body, and supports weight loss. The blend of tomatoes, celery, and basil provides essential nutrients that help boost metabolism, making it a perfect addition to a healthy diet. By choosing this juice, you are making a conscious decision to nourish your body and support your health goals.

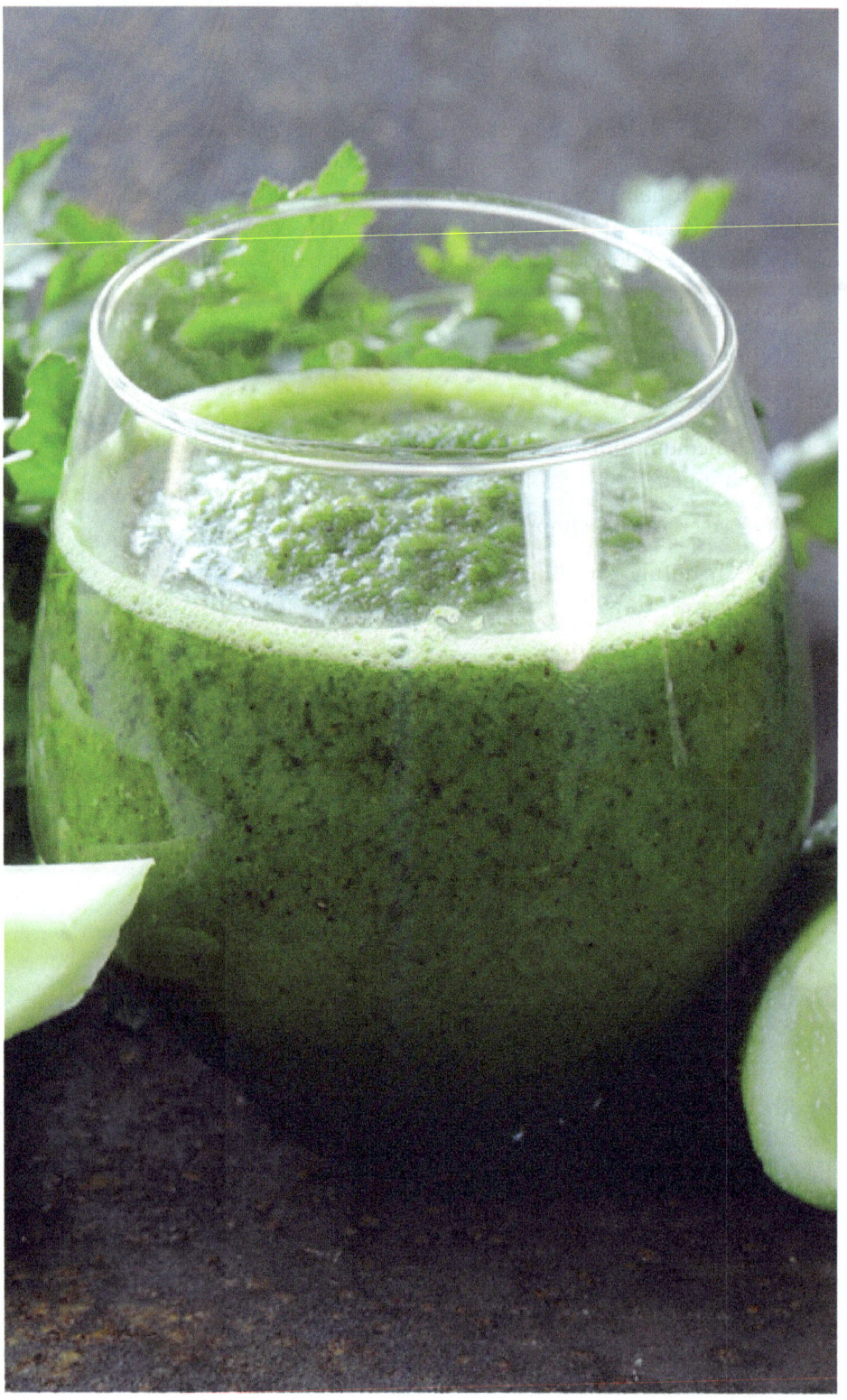

Herb Garden Juice

Fresh Green Juice, made from celery, cucumbers, and parsley, is not just a delicious drink, but also a powerhouse of health benefits. It is a hydrating and detoxifying drink that supports weight loss. Packed with vitamins, minerals, and antioxidants, this low-calorie juice boosts metabolism, helps flush out toxins, and keeps you full. It is a refreshing, light drink that fits perfectly into a healthy diet.

Servings: 1

Prepping Time: 5 minutes

Cook Time: 0 minutes

Difficulty: Easy

Ingredients:

- ✓ 2 celery stalks, chopped
- ✓ 1 cucumber, peeled and chopped
- ✓ A handful of fresh parsley
- ✓ 1/2 lemon, juiced
- ✓ 1/2 cup water
- ✓ Ice cubes (optional)

Step-by-Step Preparation:

1. Place celery, cucumber, and parsley in a blender with water.
2. Blend until smooth.
3. Strain the mixture to remove the pulp if preferred.
4. Stir in lemon juice and serve over ice if desired.

Nutritional Facts (Per serving):

- ❖ **Calories**: 40
- ❖ **Protein**: 1g
- ❖ **Fiber**: 2g
- ❖ **Carbs**: 9g
- ❖ **Fat**: 0g

This fresh green juice is a nutrient-dense, low-calorie drink that helps detoxify and rehydrate the body. It's refreshing taste and health benefits aid digestion and support weight loss, making it a great option for a healthy daily routine.

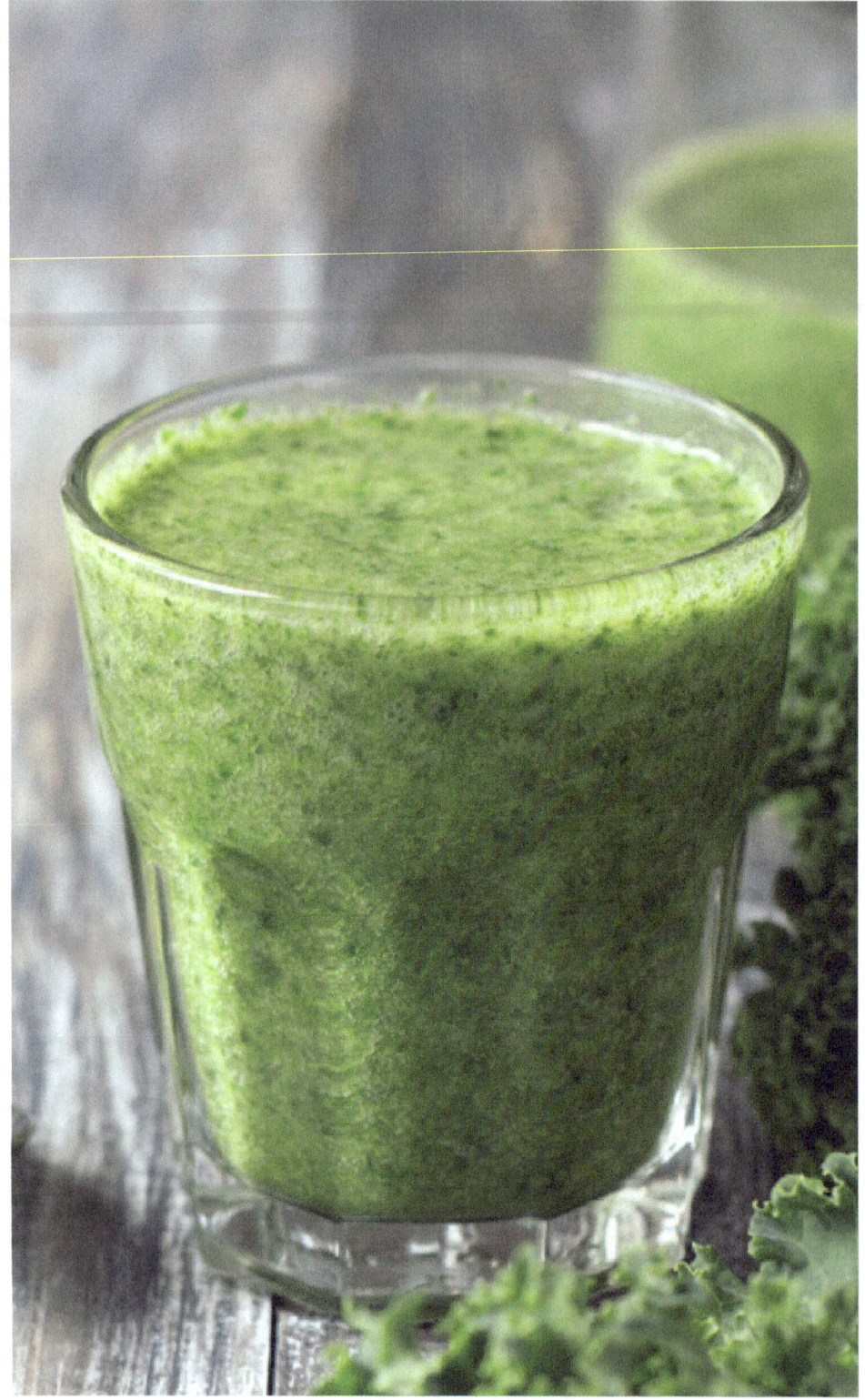

Green Smoothies With Kale, Banana and Lemon

Green Smoothies with kale, banana, and lemon offer a perfect balance of nutrition and taste for weight loss. This vibrant smoothie is not only rich in fiber, vitamins, and antioxidants, but also delicious. The combination of nutrient-dense kale, creamy banana, and zesty lemon makes it an energizing and satisfying drink for any time of the day.

Servings: 1

Cook Time: 0 minutes

Prepping Time: 5 minutes

Difficulty: Easy

Ingredients:

- ✓ 1 cup kale, chopped
- ✓ 1 ripe banana
- ✓ 1/2 lemon, juiced
- ✓ 1/2 cup water
- ✓ Ice cubes (optional)

Step-by-Step Preparation:

1. Add kale, banana, lemon juice, and water to a blender.
2. Blend until smooth and creamy.
3. Add ice cubes if desired, and blend again for a chilled smoothie.
4. Pour into a glass and serve immediately.

Nutritional Facts (Per serving):

- ❖ **Calories**: 120
- ❖ **Carbs**: 30g
- ❖ **Protein**: 2g
- ❖ **Fat**: 0g
- ❖ **Fiber**: 5g

This green smoothie is not just a delicious treat, but a powerful tool to support your health and weight loss journey. Packed with essential nutrients, it aids digestion, detoxifies your body, and provides natural energy to keep you feeling refreshed and motivated throughout the day.

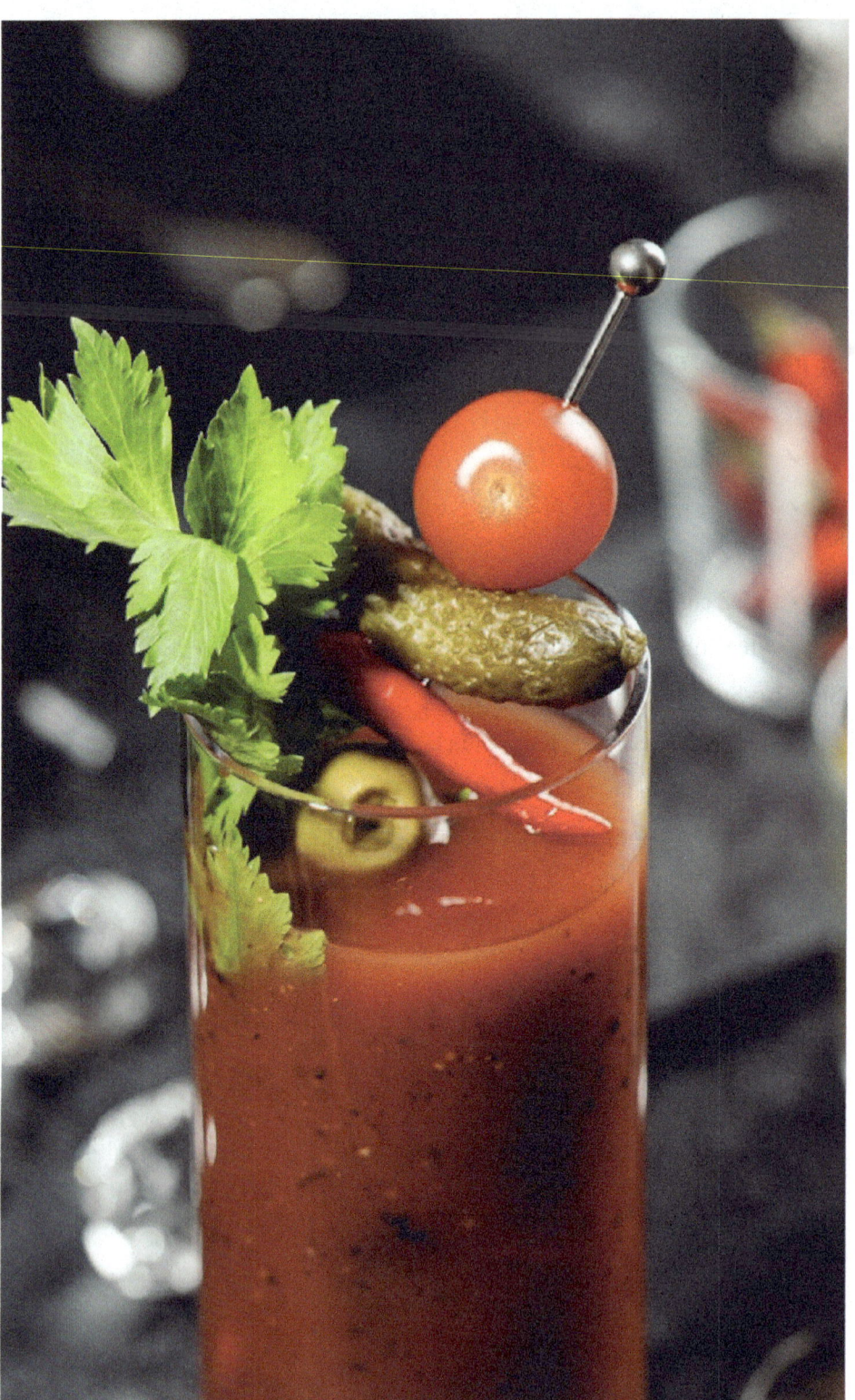

Bloody Mary Cocktail

Looking for a refreshing, savory juice to help with weight loss? This Bloody Mary cocktail mix with celery, pickle, olive, and red pepper is a tangy and nutritious drink for any time of the day. It is a perfect choice for those on a weight loss journey.

Servings: 1

Cook Time: 0 minutes

Prepping Time: 5 minutes

Difficulty: Easy

Ingredients:

- ✓ 1 cup tomato juice
- ✓ 1 celery stalk
- ✓ 1 pickle
- ✓ 2 olives
- ✓ 1 red pepper
- ✓ 1 tsp lemon juice
- ✓ 1 dash of hot sauce (optional)

Step-by-Step Preparation:

1. Wash the celery, pickle, olive, and red pepper.
2. Blend all ingredients until smooth.
3. Pour into a glass and enjoy!

Nutritional Facts: *(Per serving)*

- ❖ **Calories:** 40
- ❖ **Fiber:** 3g
- ❖ **Protein:** 2g
- ❖ **Fat:** 1g
- ❖ **Carbs:** 8g

Perfect for a light, low-calorie refreshment, this cocktail mix helps you stay on track with your health goals while offering a satisfying, savory flavor. Enjoy it chilled for maximum freshness!

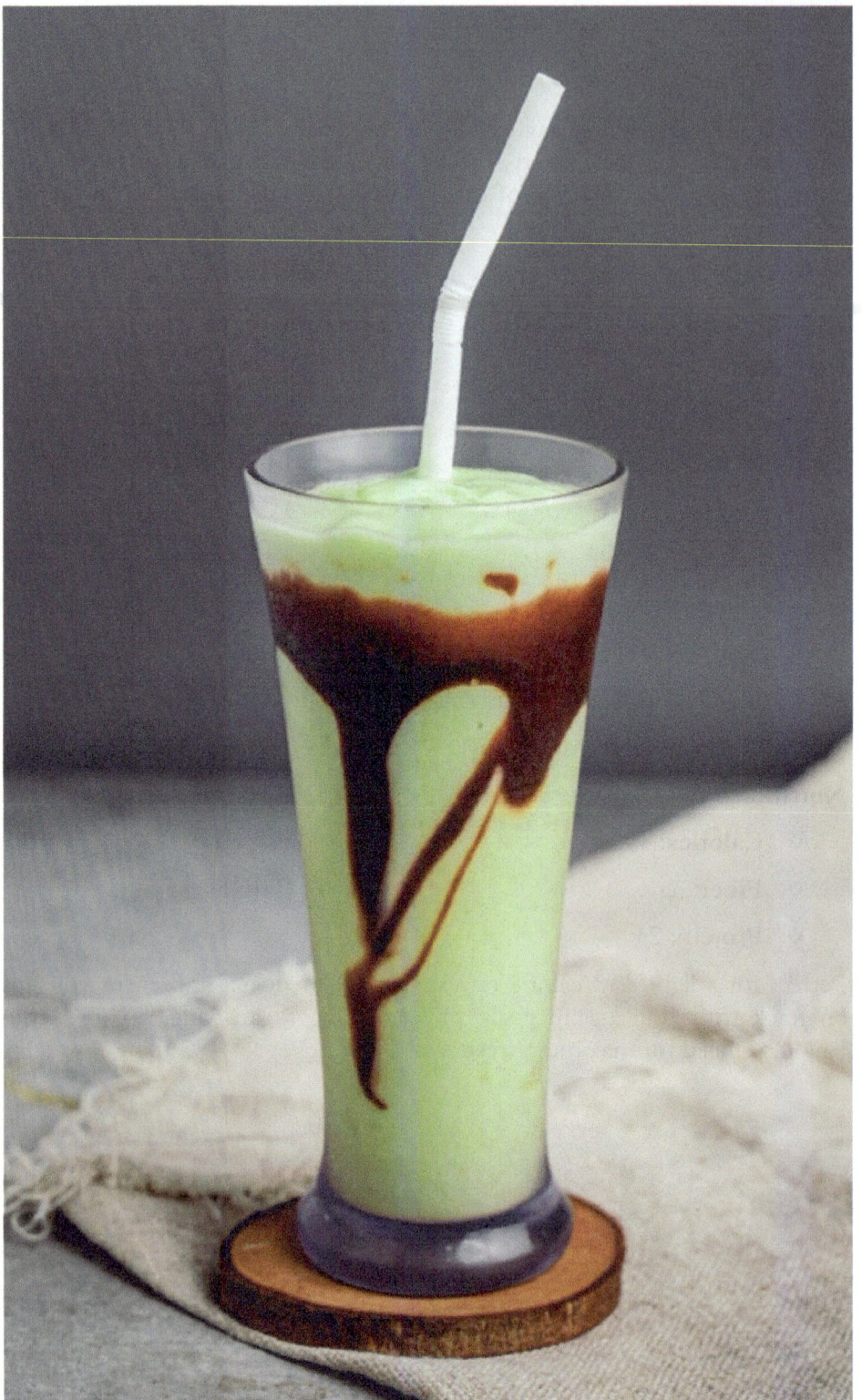

Avocado Juice With Chocolate Syrup

Craving a creamy yet healthy treat? This avocado juice with chocolate syrup is a tantalizing blend of rich flavors and weight loss benefits. The smooth avocado provides healthy fats, while the chocolate syrup adds a touch of indulgence, creating a delicious and balanced taste experience.

Servings: 1

Cook Time: 0 minutes

Prepping Time: 5 minutes

Difficulty: Easy

Ingredients:

- ✓ 1 ripe avocado
- ✓ 1 cup almond milk
- ✓ 1 tbsp chocolate syrup (sugar-free, optional)
- ✓ 1 tsp honey (optional)
- ✓ Ice cubes

Step-by-Step Preparation:

1. Scoop the avocado into a blender.
2. Add almond milk, chocolate syrup, honey, and ice cubes.
3. Blend until smooth and creamy.
4. Pour into a glass and enjoy chilled!

Nutritional Facts: *(Per serving)*

- ❖ **Calories:** 180
- ❖ **Fat:** 15g
- ❖ **Fiber:** 7g
- ❖ **Carbs:** 12g
- ❖ **Protein:** 3g

Indulge in this rich and satisfying juice, which not only delights your taste buds but also energizes you. Its creamy texture and subtle sweetness make it a delightful treat for weight loss.

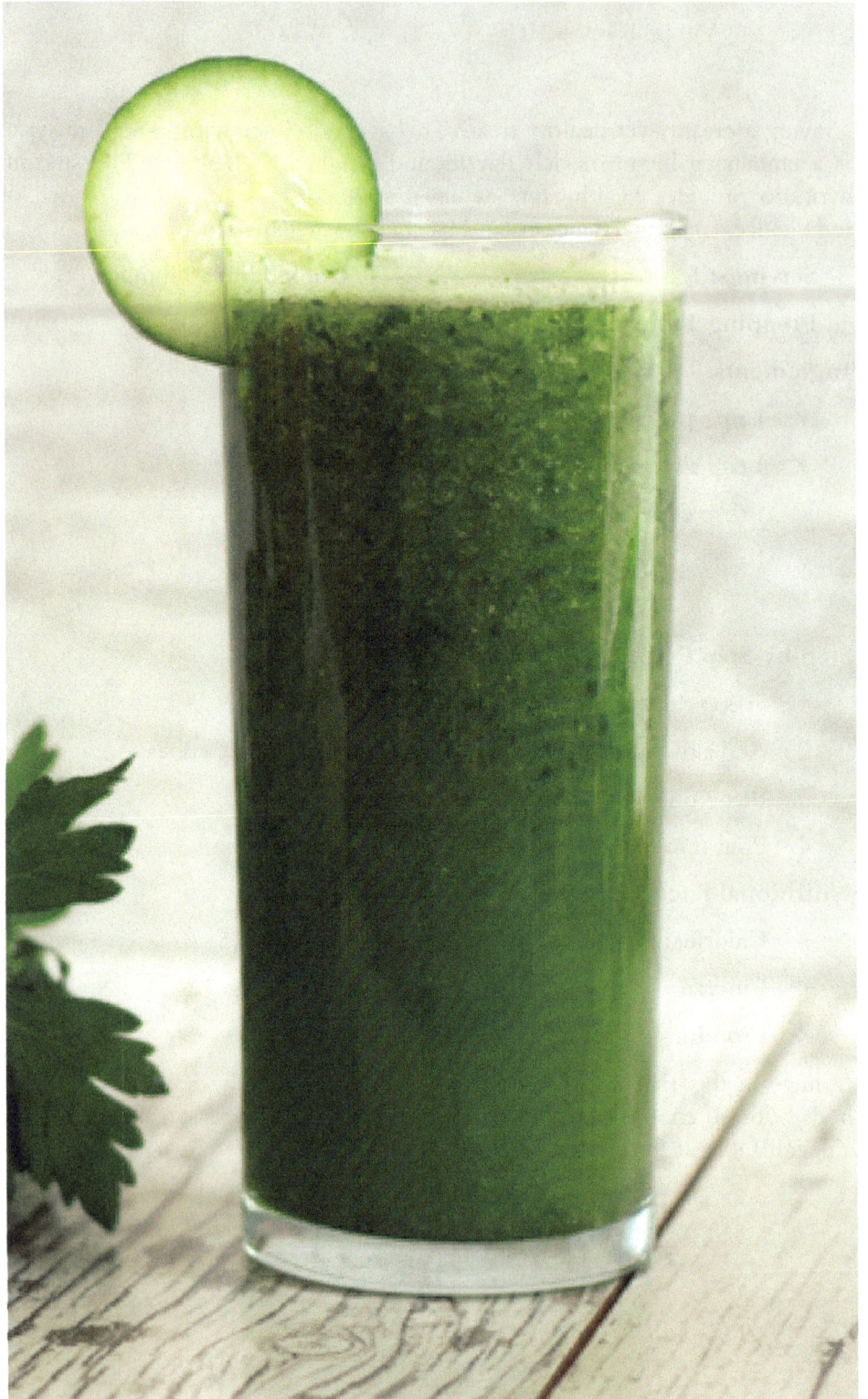

Parsley Power Boost

Looking for a refreshing, detoxifying juice to aid in weight loss? This green juice made with cucumber, lemon, and parsley is a powerhouse of hydration, vitamins, and antioxidants. It is not just a tasty drink, but a health-boosting elixir that can cleanse your body and keep you energized.

Servings: 1

Cook Time: 0 minutes

Prepping Time: 5 minutes

Difficulty: Easy

Ingredients:

- ✓ 1 cucumber
- ✓ 1/2 lemon (juiced)
- ✓ A handful of fresh parsley
- ✓ 1 cup water
- ✓ Ice cubes

Step-by-Step Preparation:

1. Peel and chop the cucumber.
2. Add cucumber, lemon juice, parsley, and water to a blender.
3. Blend until smooth.
4. Strain if desired and serve chilled over ice.

Nutritional Facts: *(Per serving)*

- ❖ **Calories:** 30
- ❖ **Fat:** 0g
- ❖ **Fiber:** 2g
- ❖ **Carbs:** 6g
- ❖ **Protein:** 1g

Before starting any weight loss regimen, it is important to consult a healthcare professional. This light, detoxifying juice is perfect for a refreshing pick-me-up. It aids digestion and promotes hydration. Enjoy this natural cleanser anytime to refresh and revitalize your weight loss journey.

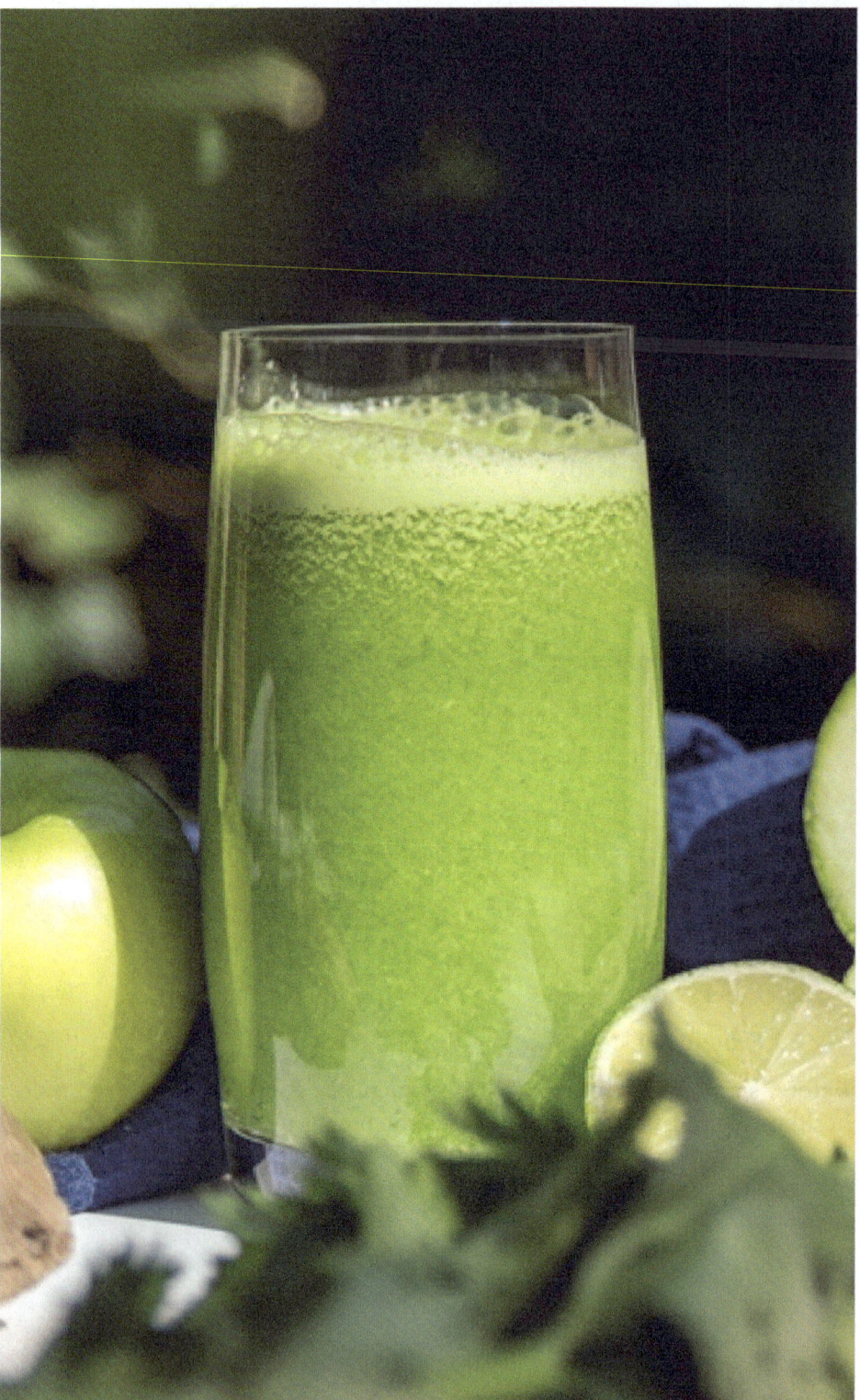

Zesty Veggie Medley

Indulge in a refreshing green smoothie made with cucumber, zucchini, basil, apple, and ginger. This nutrient-packed drink is not only perfect for enjoying amidst nature, but also aids in weight loss. It provides a revitalizing blend of flavors to kickstart your day, while the health benefits of the ingredients will leave you feeling reassured about your dietary choices.

Servings: 1

Cook Time: 0 minutes

Prepping Time: 5 minutes

Difficulty: Easy

Ingredients:

- ✓ 1 cucumber
- ✓ 1/2 zucchini
- ✓ 1 green apple
- ✓ A handful of fresh basil
- ✓ 1/2-inch ginger
- ✓ 1 cup water
- ✓ Ice cubes

Step-by-Step Preparation:

1. Peel and chop the cucumber, zucchini, and apple.
2. Add all ingredients to a blender, along with water and ginger.
3. Blend until smooth and creamy.
4. Serve chilled with ice and enjoy.

Nutritional Facts: *(Per serving)*

- ❖ **Calories:** 70
- ❖ **Fiber:** 4g
- ❖ **Protein:** 2g
- ❖ **Fat:** 0g
- ❖ **Carbs:** 15g

This refreshing smoothie is perfect for sipping while surrounded by nature. It is a delightful combination of greens and fruit, giving you the right balance of nutrients to fuel your weight loss journey while keeping you hydrated and satisfied.

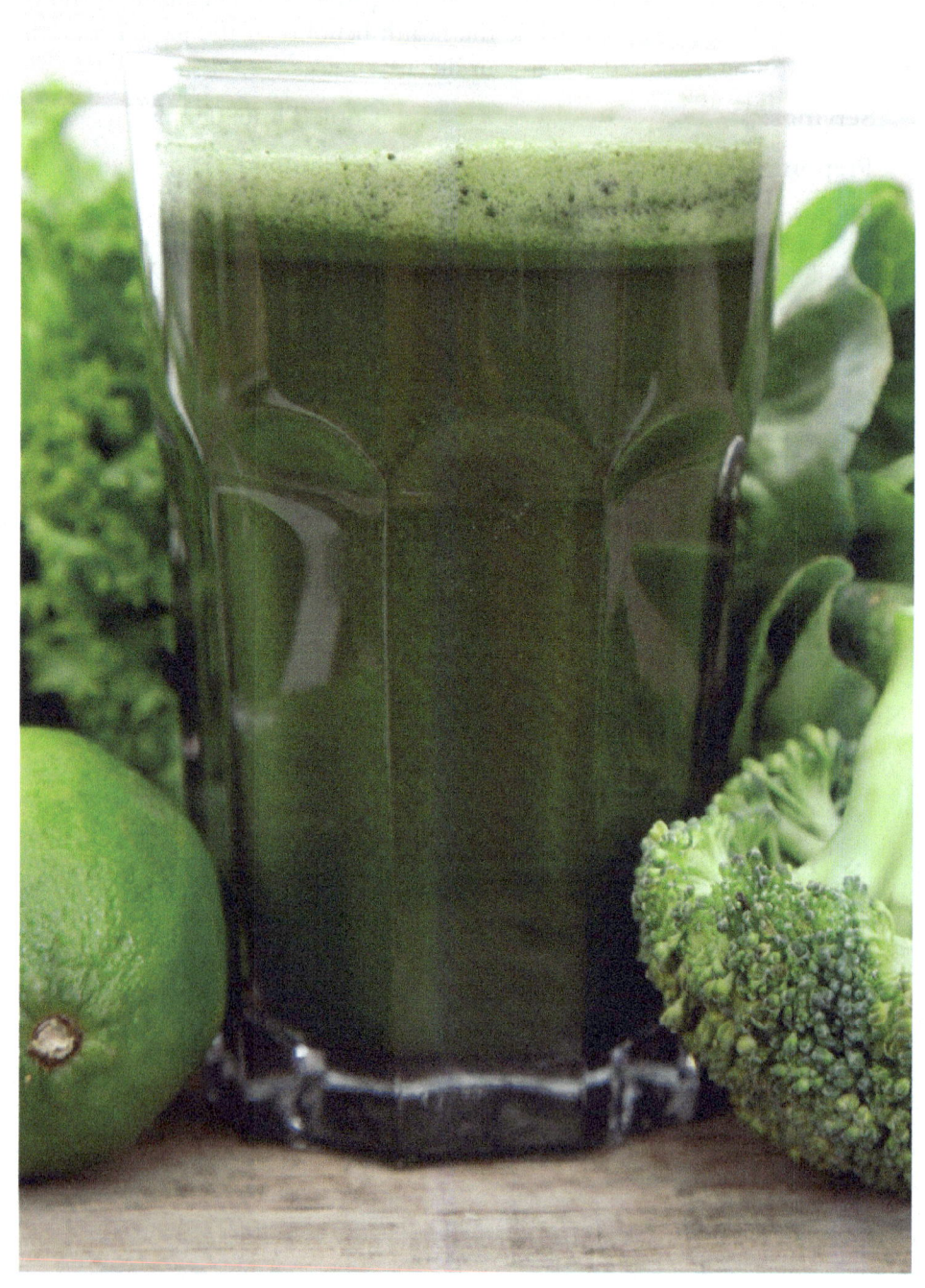

Boost your weight loss journey with this nutrient-dense broccoli juice blended with spinach, parsley, and lemon. This refreshing green drink is packed with vitamins and antioxidants, making it the perfect detox juice to fuel your body and promote overall well-being.

Servings: 1   **Cook Time:** 0 minutes

Prepping Time: 5 minutes   **Difficulty:** Easy

Ingredients:

- ✓ 1/2 cup broccoli florets
- ✓ 1 handful spinach
- ✓ A handful of fresh parsley
- ✓ 1/2 lemon (juiced)
- ✓ 1 cup water
- ✓ Ice cubes

Step-by-Step Preparation:

1. Rinse the broccoli, spinach, and parsley.
2. Blend all ingredients with water until smooth.
3. Strain if needed, and serve over ice.

Nutritional Facts: *(Per serving)*

- ❖ **Calories:** 40
- ❖ **Fiber:** 3g
- ❖ **Protein:** 3g
- ❖ **Fat:** 0g
- ❖ **Carbs:** 8g

This detoxifying juice is more than just a refreshing burst of nutrients. It's a powerful energizer that can kickstart your metabolism and keep you invigorated throughout the day, helping you stay on track with your weight loss goals.

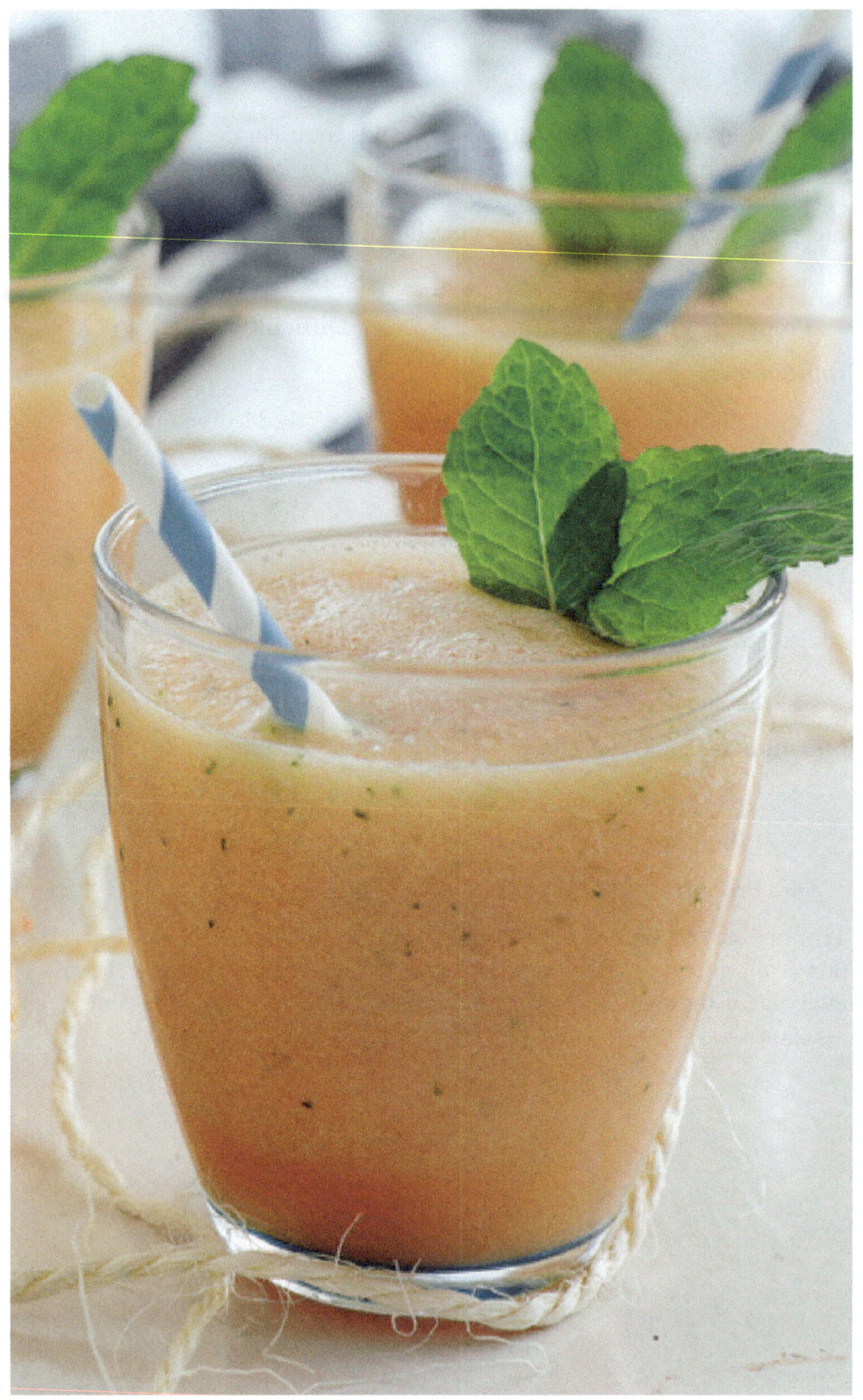

Weight Loss Juices

Fat Burner Delight

Looking for a fat-burning boost? This delightful juice made with grapefruit, pineapple, and lemon not only has metabolism-boosting properties but also provides a refreshing burst of citrus flavors. It is the perfect drink to support your weight loss goals while keeping you hydrated and energized.

Servings: 1

Prepping Time: 5 minutes

Cook Time: 0 minutes

Difficulty: Easy

Ingredients:

- ✓ 1/2 grapefruit (juiced)
- ✓ 1/2 cup pineapple chunks
- ✓ 1/2 lemon (juiced)
- ✓ 1 cup water
- ✓ Ice cubes

Step-by-Step Preparation:

1. Juice the grapefruit and lemon.
2. Add the pineapple chunks, juices, and water to a blender.
3. Blend until smooth, and serve over ice.

Nutritional Facts: *(Per serving)*

- ❖ **Calories:** 60
- ❖ **Fiber:** 2g
- ❖ **Protein:** 1g
- ❖ **Fat:** 0g
- ❖ **Carbs:** 14g

Enjoy this fat-burning delight as a refreshing way to kickstart your metabolism and boost energy. The perfect blend of tangy and sweet, this juice is a satisfying companion for your weight loss journey, helping you feel refreshed and invigorated.

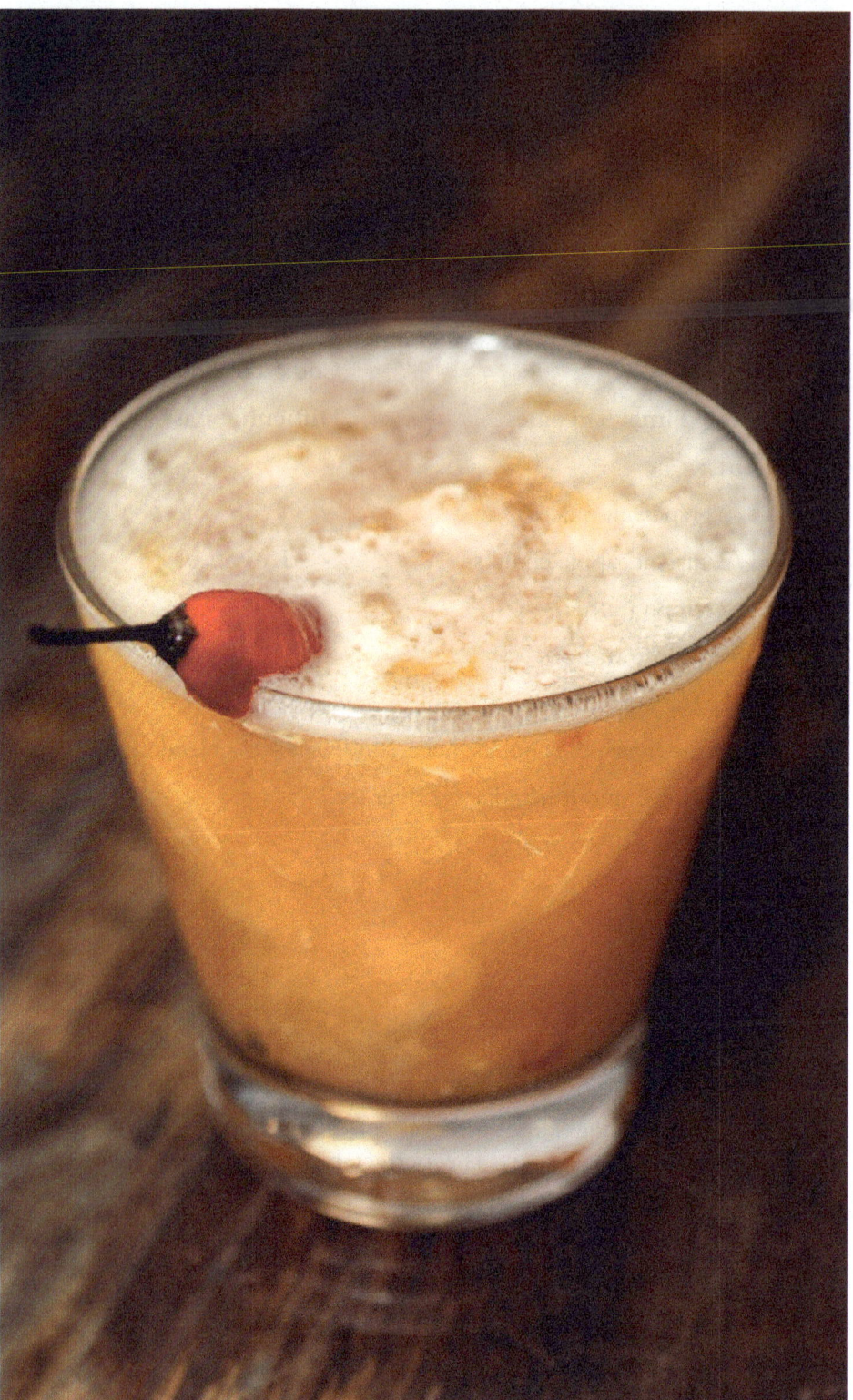

Metabolism Boosting Tonic

Boost your metabolism and your health with this zesty tonic made from lemon, ginger, and cayenne. These ingredients are known for their fat-burning and detoxifying properties, and when combined, they create a potent, refreshing drink. This tonic not only enhances digestion and boosts energy but also supports your weight loss efforts, making it a great addition to your health routine.

Servings: 1

Prepping Time: 5 minutes

Cook Time: 0 minutes

Difficulty: Easy

Ingredients:

- ✓ 1/2 lemon (juiced)
- ✓ 1/2-inch piece of fresh ginger
- ✓ 1 pinch cayenne pepper
- ✓ 1 cup water
- ✓ Ice cubes

Step-by-Step Preparation:

1. Juice the lemon and grate the ginger.
2. Add lemon juice, ginger, cayenne, and water to a blender.
3. Blend well and serve over ice.

Nutritional Facts: *(Per serving)*

- ❖ **Calories:** 10
- ❖ **Fiber:** 0g
- ❖ **Protein:** 0g
- ❖ **Fat:** 0g
- ❖ **Carbs:** 2g

This metabolism-boosting tonic is more than just a drink. It is a burst of energy that cleanses and refreshes your system. It is the perfect way to kickstart your day or give yourself a mid-afternoon boost. With its fiery kick, it is both invigorating and satisfying. Enjoy it as a morning boost or an afternoon pick-me-up!

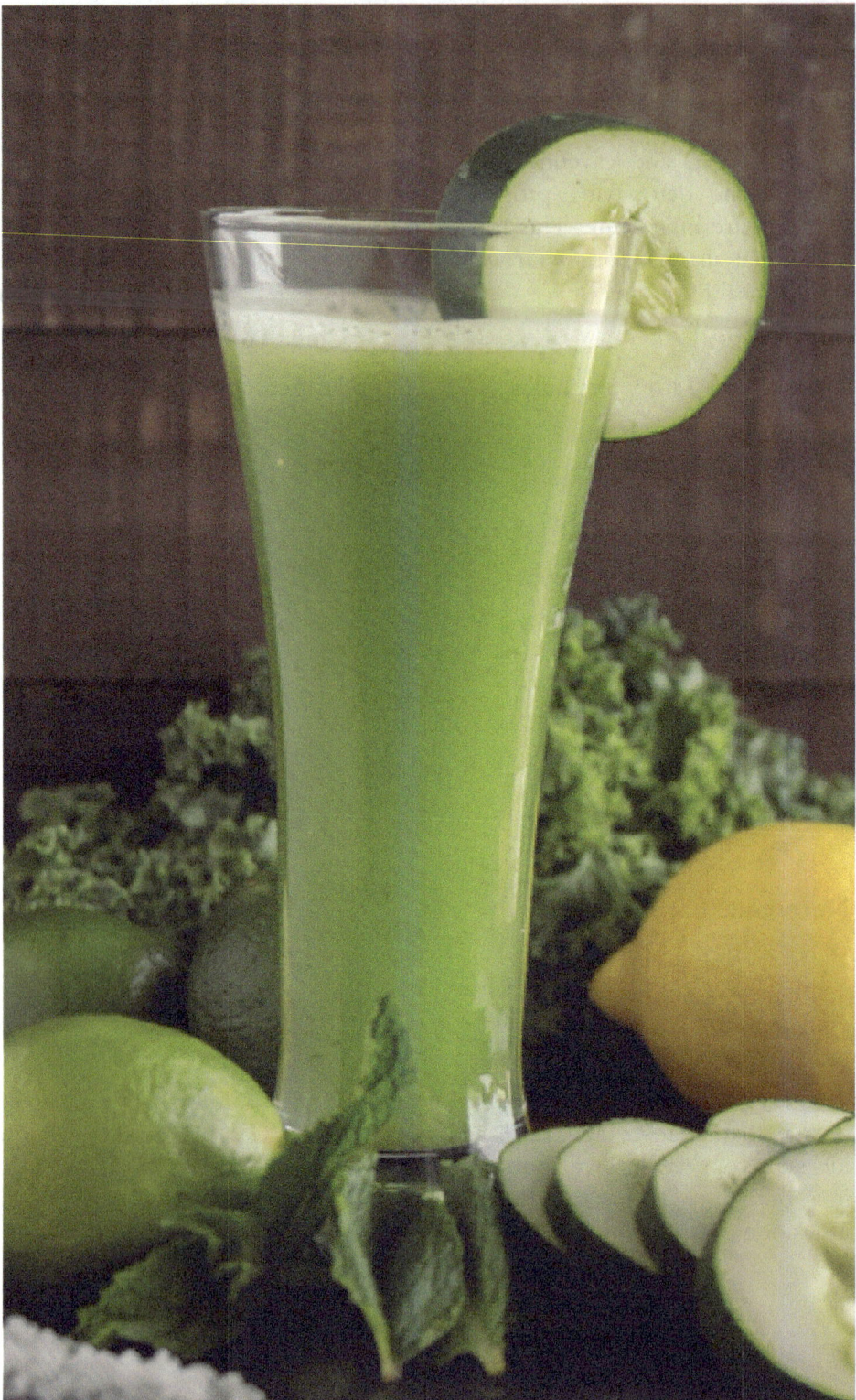

Slim Down Super Juice

Refresh your weight loss journey with this Slim Down Super Juice made from cucumber, lemon, and mint. This hydrating and detoxifying blend not only helps flush out toxins and boost digestion but also provides a refreshing burst of energy, making it an ideal drink for shedding those extra pounds and keeping you invigorated throughout the day.

Servings: 1

Cook Time: 0 minutes

Prepping Time: 5 minutes

Difficulty: Easy

Ingredients:

- ✓ 1 cucumber
- ✓ 1/2 lemon (juiced)
- ✓ A handful of fresh mint leaves
- ✓ 1 cup water
- ✓ Ice cubes

Step-by-Step Preparation:

1. Peel and chop the cucumber.
2. Add cucumber, lemon juice, mint, and water to a blender.
3. Blend until smooth, and serve over ice.

Nutritional Facts: *(Per serving)*

- ❖ **Calories:** 20
- ❖ **Fiber:** 2g
- ❖ **Protein:** 1g
- ❖ **Fat:** 0g
- ❖ **Carbs:** 4g

This light and refreshing juice is not only perfect for weight loss goals, but also for your overall health. The excellent combination of cucumber, lemon, and mint helps hydrate and cleanse your system, giving you a revitalizing boost throughout the day. Sip and slim down with ease, knowing that you are nourishing your body with every sip.

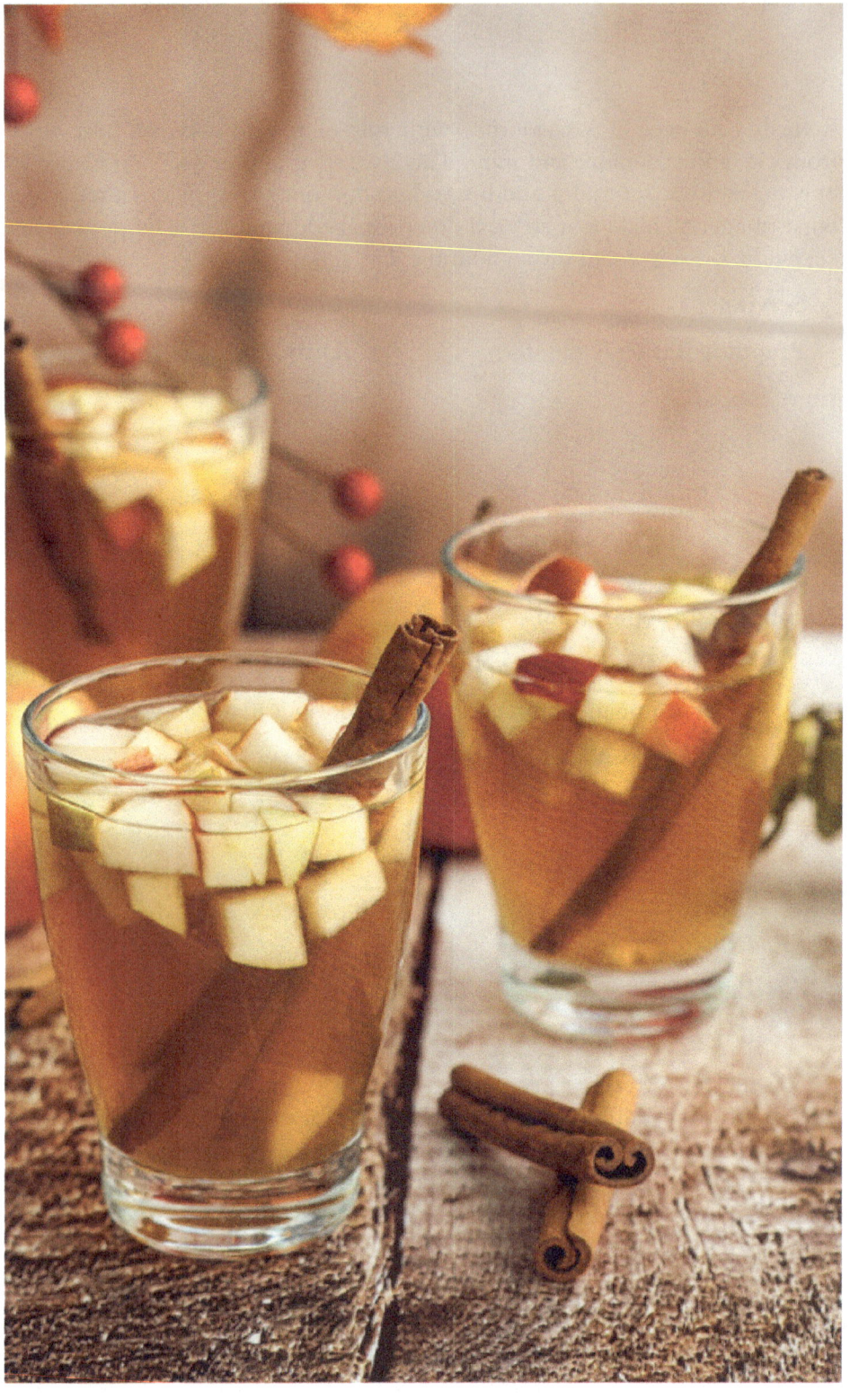

Apple Cinnamon Slimmer

Enjoy this delicious **Apple Cinnamon Slimmer** juice, perfect for weight loss and packed with refreshing flavors. Combining apples, pears, and cinnamon, it is a nutritious, fat-burning drink to kickstart your day.

Servings: 2

Prepping Time: 10 minutes

Cook Time: 0 minutes

Difficulty: Easy

Ingredients:

- ✓ 2 apples
- ✓ 2 pears
- ✓ 1/2 teaspoon cinnamon
- ✓ Ice cubes (optional)

Step-by-Step Preparation:

1. Core and chop apples and pears.
2. Add them to a juicer.
3. Sprinkle cinnamon on top.
4. Blend until smooth.
5. Serve with ice if desired.

Nutritional Facts: (Per serving)

- ❖ **Calories:** 100
- ❖ **Carbs:** 25g
- ❖ **Fiber:** 5g
- ❖ **Protein:** 1g

By sipping this refreshing juice regularly, you are not just enjoying a delicious drink, but also promoting weight loss in a natural way. Packed with vitamins and fiber, it is the perfect mid-morning refreshment to keep you energized and on tracks with your health goals.

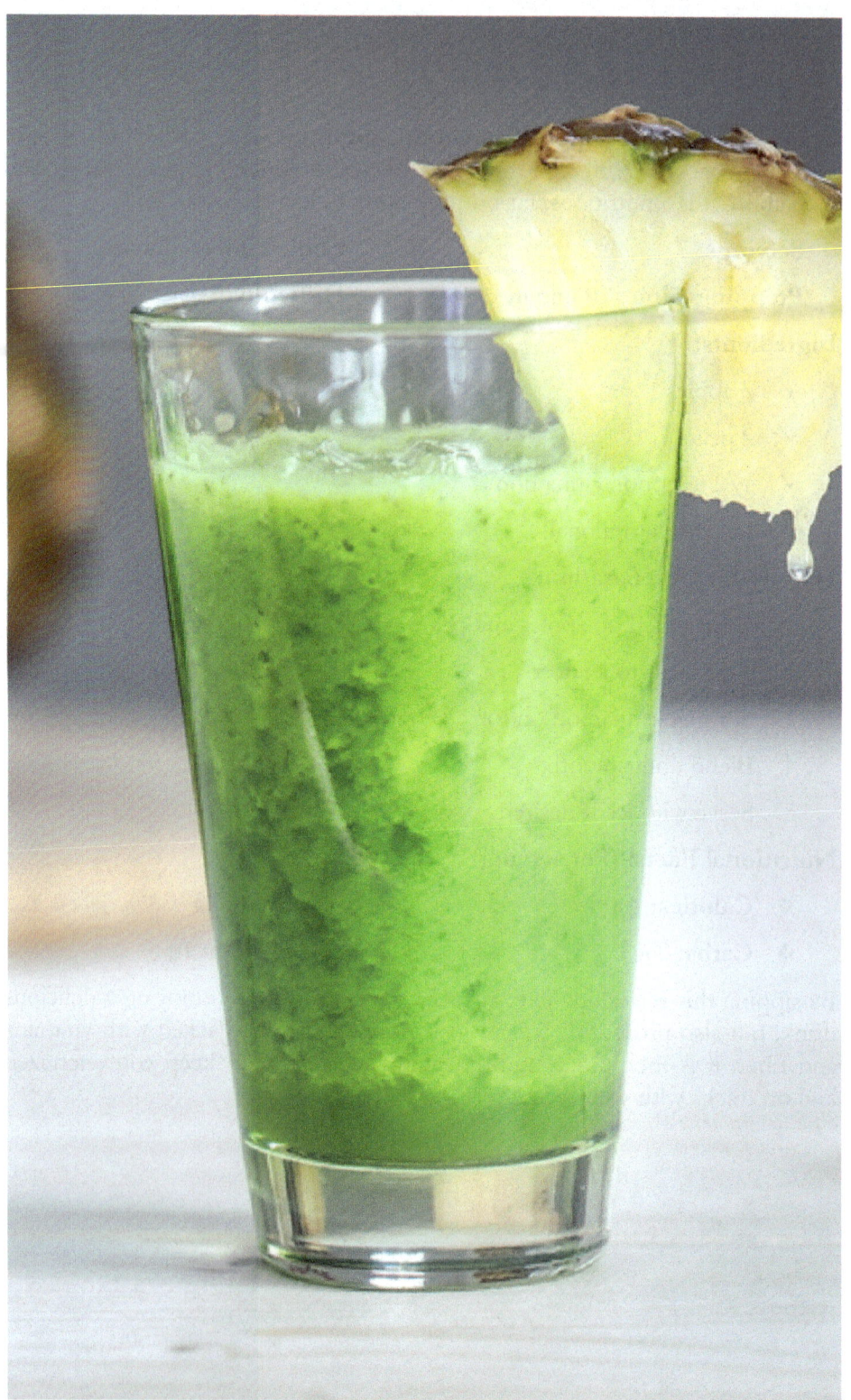

Pineapple Detox Slimmer

This refreshing **Pineapple Detox Slimmer** juice is not just a delicious drink, but also a powerful tool for weight loss and cleansing. Packed with the goodness of pineapple, lemon, and cucumber, it is a hydrating, nutrient-packed elixir that boosts metabolism and detoxifies your body. Knowing that each sip is contributing to your health and wellness can be a great motivator.

Servings: 1

Cook Time: 0 minutes

Prepping Time: 5 minutes

Difficulty: Easy

Ingredients:

- ✓ 1/2 pineapple, peeled and chopped
- ✓ 1/2 cucumber
- ✓ 1/2 lemon, juiced
- ✓ Ice cubes (optional)

Step-by-Step Preparation:

1. Chop pineapple and cucumber.
2. Add them to a juicer.
3. Squeeze lemon juice into the mix.
4. Blend until smooth.
5. Serve chilled with ice.

Nutritional Facts: (Per serving)

- ❖ **Calories:** 90
- ❖ **Fiber:** 4g
- ❖ **Carbs:** 22g
- ❖ **Protein:** 1g

This light and tasty juice is perfect for a detox boost. Its blend of fruits and veggies will energize you, refresh you, and get you ready to shed some pounds!

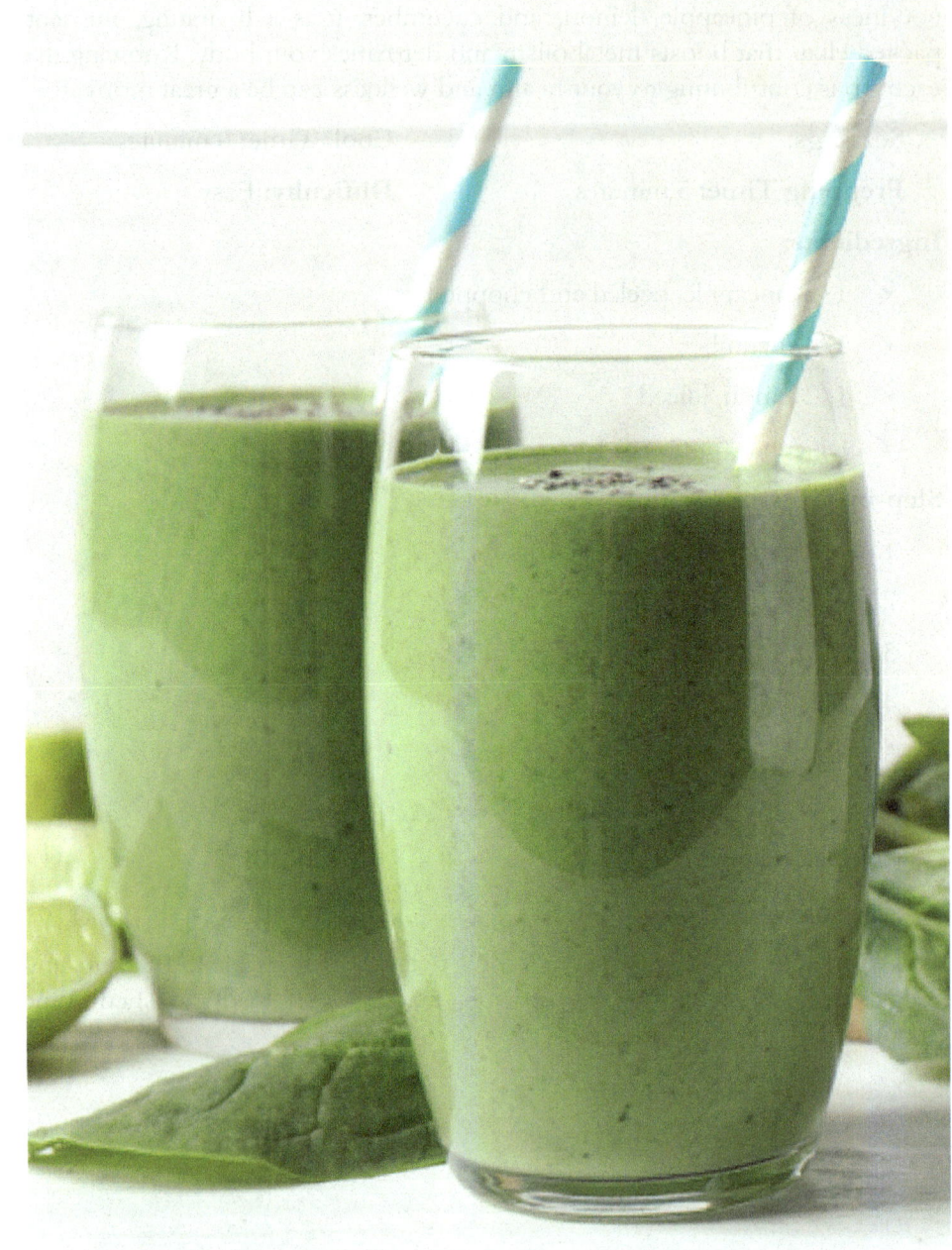

Green Juices

Cucumber Lime Refreshment

This **Cucumber Lime Refreshment** is a revitalizing weight-loss juice made with natural, hydrating cucumber, zesty lime, and nutrient-packed spinach. It refreshes you while supporting your weight-loss goals, perfect for a detox boost. With these natural ingredients, you can feel connected to the recipe and the health benefits it offers.

Servings: 2

Prepping Time: 5 minutes

Cook Time: 0 minutes

Difficulty: Easy

Ingredients:

- ✓ 2 cucumbers, peeled and chopped
- ✓ 1 lime, juiced
- ✓ 1 cup fresh spinach
- ✓ Ice cubes (optional)

Step-by-Step Preparation:

1. Chop cucumbers and add to a juicer.
2. Add fresh spinach leaves.
3. Squeeze lime juice into the mix.
4. Blend until smooth, then serve with ice if desired.

Nutritional Facts: (Per serving)

- ❖ **Calories:** 35
- ❖ **Carbs:** 8g
- ❖ **Fiber:** 2g
- ❖ **Protein:** 1g

This refreshing juice is not just a tasty drink, but also an excellent way to stay hydrated and cleanse your body naturally. The mix of cucumber, lime, and spinach makes it a low-calorie drink that boosts metabolism and supports weight loss, giving you the reassurance that you are making a healthy choice.

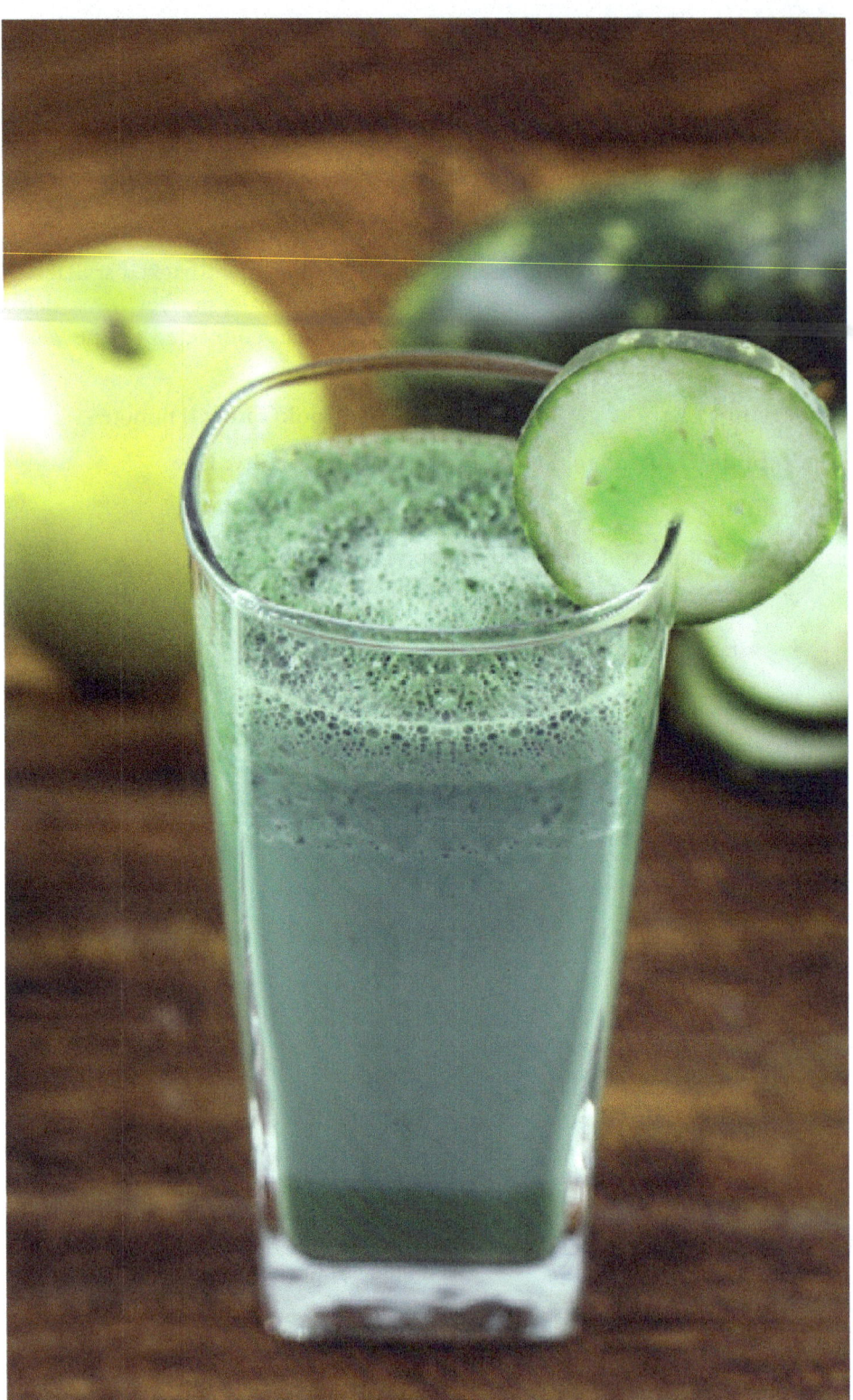

Kale Lemon Kick

The **Kale Lemon Kick** is a nutrient-rich, detoxifying juice perfect for weight loss. Its ingredients include kale, lemon, apple, lettuce, cucumber, and lime. This refreshing drink is packed with antioxidants and vitamins to boost your metabolism and energy levels.

Servings: 1

Cook Time: 0 minutes

Prepping Time: 5 minutes

Difficulty: Easy

Ingredients:

- ✓ 1 cup kale leaves
- ✓ 1/2 lemon, juiced
- ✓ 1 apple, chopped
- ✓ 1/2 cup lettuce leaves
- ✓ 1/2 cucumber, chopped
- ✓ 1/2 lime, juiced

Step-by-Step Preparation:

1. Add kale, apple, lettuce, and cucumber to the juicer.
2. Squeeze in the lemon and lime juices.
3. Blend until smooth.
4. Serve chilled with ice if desired.

Nutritional Facts: (Per serving)

- ❖ **Calories:** 60
- ❖ **Fiber:** 4g
- ❖ **Carbs:** 15g
- ❖ **Protein:** 2g

This **Kale Lemon Kick** is not just a delicious drink, it's a powerhouse of nutrients. It is ideal for detoxifying and aiding in weight loss. Enjoy this tangy, refreshing juice as a light, healthy snack or meal replacement to energize you throughout the day. Knowing that you are nourishing your body with every sip can be a great motivator on your health journey.

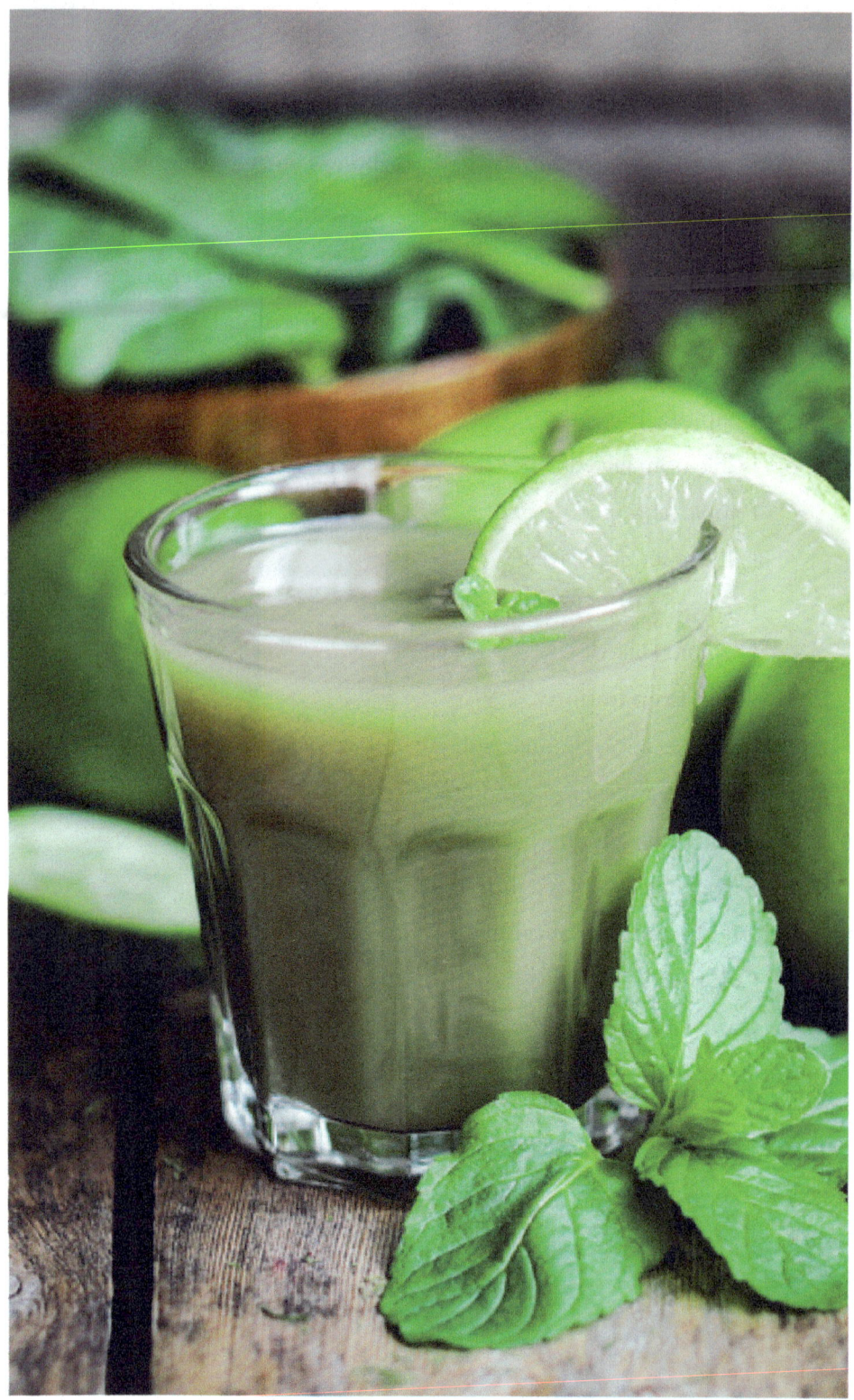

Minty Green Energizer

This refreshing minty green energizer is not just a weight loss boost but also a natural energy source. It is made with cucumber, mint, and green apple, all of which are packed with hydrating ingredients and natural energy. This juice is a light, invigorating, and nutrient-dense choice that will keep you going and provide a healthy boost to your day.

Servings: 1

Cook Time: 0 minutes

Prepping Time: 5 minutes

Difficulty: Easy

Ingredients:

- ✓ 1 cucumber
- ✓ 1 green apple
- ✓ A handful of fresh mint leaves
- ✓ ½ lemon (juiced)
- ✓ ½ cup cold water (optional)

Step-by-Step Preparation:

1. Wash all produce thoroughly.
2. Cut the cucumber and green apple into pieces.
3. Add cucumber, apple, mint, and lemon juice to a juicer.
4. Juice until smooth; add cold water if desired.
5. Pour into a glass and serve chilled.

Nutritional Facts (Per serving):

- ❖ **Calories**: 90
- ❖ **Sugar**: 15g
- ❖ **Carbs**: 22g
- ❖ **Vitamin C**: 30%
- ❖ **Fiber**: 4g

Enjoy this light, minty juice as a refreshing addition to your weight loss journey. The cucumber hydrates, while the mint and apple provide flavor and essential nutrients. Feel energized and nourished with each sip!

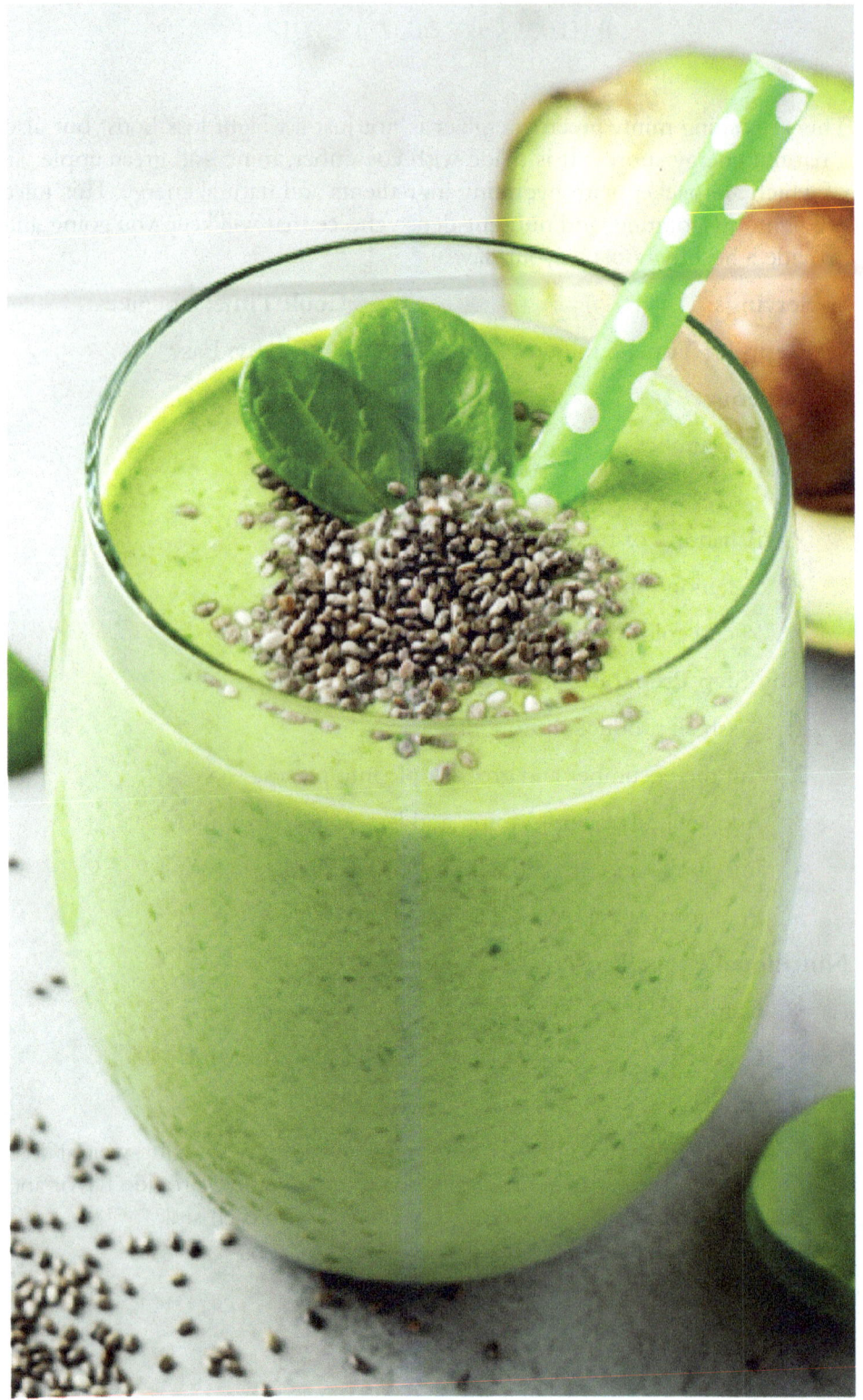

Avocado Spinach Dream

This creamy Avocado Spinach Dream juice is a perfect choice for weight loss. It combines the healthy fats of avocado with nutrient-rich spinach, apple, and chia seeds. It is a refreshing yet filling drink that helps keep hunger at bay while providing essential nutrients for your weight loss journey.

Servings: 1

Prepping Time: 5 minutes

Cook Time: 0 minutes

Difficulty: Easy

Ingredients:

✓ ½ avocado

✓ 1 cup fresh spinach leaves

✓ 1 apple (cored)

✓ 1 tbsp chia seeds

✓ ½ cup water

Step-by-Step Preparation:

1. Wash and prepare all ingredients.
2. Cut the avocado and apple into chunks.
3. Add avocado, spinach, apple, chia seeds, and water to a blender.
4. Blend until smooth and creamy.
5. Serve chilled in a glass.

Nutritional Facts (Per serving):

❖ **Calories**: 150

❖ **Carbs**: 24g

❖ **Fiber**: 10g

❖ **Protein**: 4g

❖ **Healthy fats**: 8g

This juice is ideal for weight loss and provides a nutrient-dense boost to your day. Fiber-rich ingredients like avocado, spinach, and chia seeds keep you feeling full while promoting healthy digestion and energy levels. Enjoy this as a wholesome snack or meal replacement!

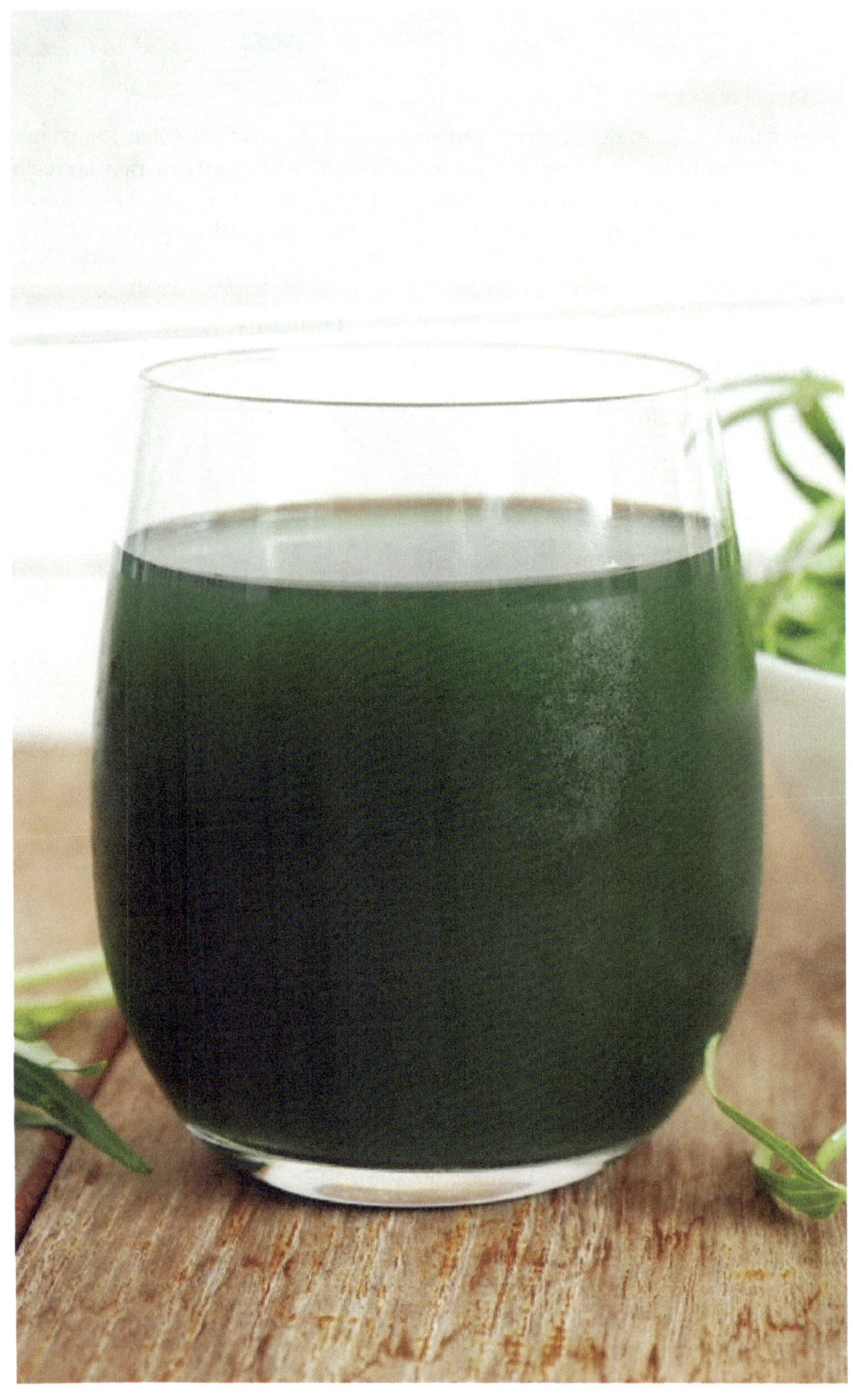

Water Spinach Sprouts Detox Juice

Water Spinach Sprouts Detox Juice is not just a refreshing, nutrient-dense drink. It is a powerhouse of vitamins, minerals, and antioxidants that can help detoxify your body and support healthy weight management. With this juice, you are not just drinking, you're nourishing your body.

Servings: 1

Prepping Time: 5 minutes

Cook Time: N/A

Difficulty: Easy

Ingredients:

- ✓ 1 cup fresh water spinach
- ✓ ½ cup sprouts
- ✓ ½ cucumber, peeled and chopped
- ✓ ½ green apple, cored and chopped
- ✓ ½ lemon, juiced
- ✓ ½ cup water

Step-by-Step Preparation:

1. Rinse and chop all ingredients.
2. Add water, spinach, sprouts, cucumber, apple, and lemon juice into a blender.
3. Blend until smooth, adding water to adjust consistency.
4. Strain the juice if desired and pour it into a glass.

Nutritional Facts (Per serving):

- ❖ **Calories**: 40
- ❖ **Carbohydrates**: 9g
- ❖ **Fiber**: 2g
- ❖ **Sugars**: 5g

Water Spinach Sprouts Detox Juice is ideal for a light and nutritious start to your day. Enjoy its detoxifying benefits and fresh taste while naturally supporting your weight loss goals with this refreshing juice.

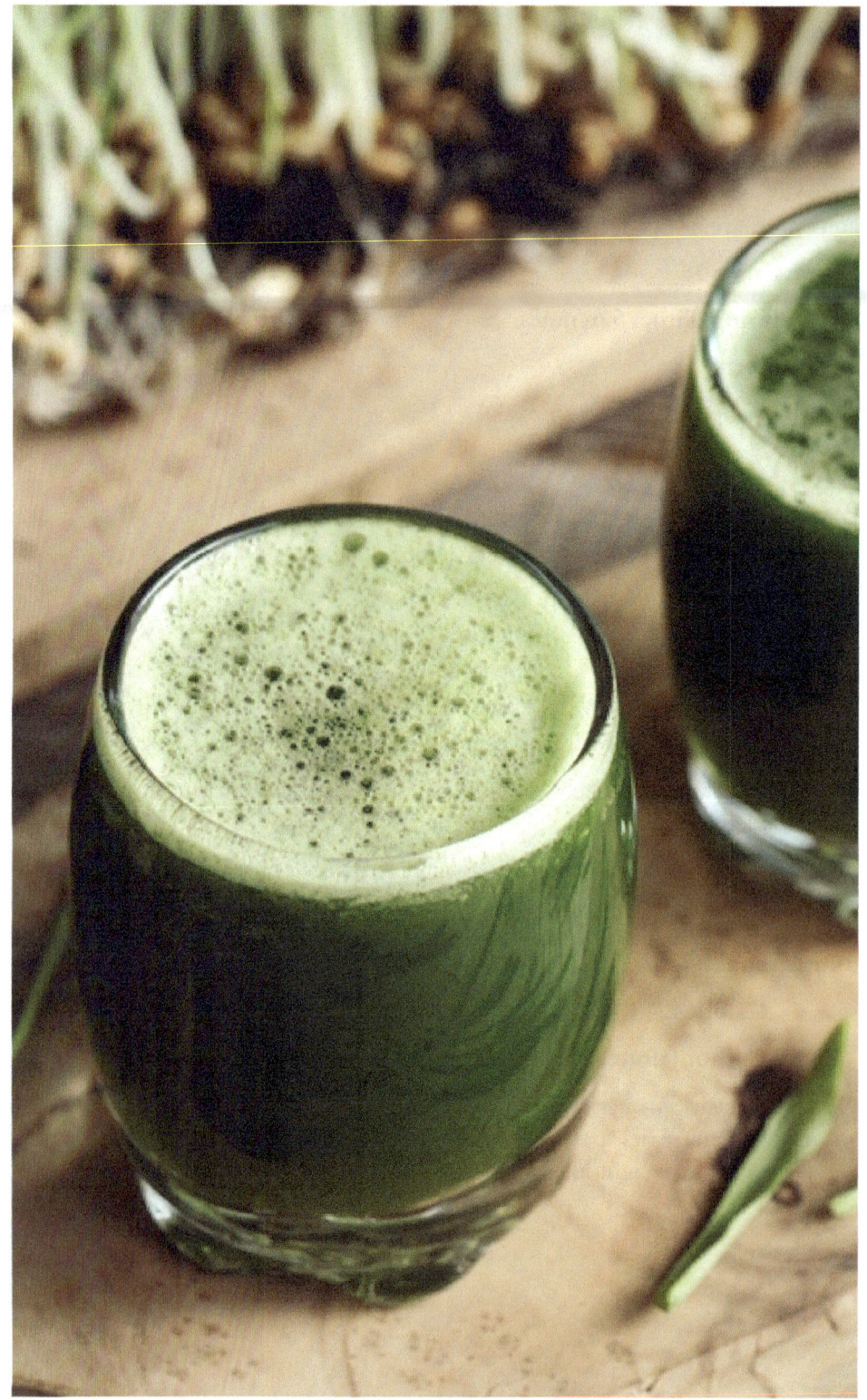

Detoxifying and Cleansing Juices

Barley Grass Juice

Barley Grass Juice is a powerhouse of nutrition, perfect for anyone looking to boost their weight loss efforts. Packed with chlorophyll, vitamins, and antioxidants, this juice aids digestion, detoxifies the body, and promotes healthy metabolism, making it a great addition to your daily routine.

Servings: 1

Prepping Time: 5 minutes

Cook Time: N/A

Difficulty: Easy

Ingredients:

- ✓ 1 tablespoon barley grass powder
- ✓ 1 cup water
- ✓ ½ cucumber, peeled and chopped
- ✓ 1 green apple, cored and chopped
- ✓ ½ lemon, juiced

Step-by-Step Preparation:

1. Add the barley grass powder to the water and stir well.
2. In a blender, combine cucumber, apple, and lemon juice.
3. Blend until smooth, then add the barley grass mixture.
4. Strain if preferred, and pour into a glass.

Nutritional Facts (Per serving):

- ❖ **Calories**: 35
- ❖ **Carbohydrates**: 8g
- ❖ **Fiber**: 2g
- ❖ **Sugars**: 5g

Barley Grass Juice is not just a simple detoxifying drink, it's a powerhouse of health-boosting properties that can support your weight loss journey. Enjoy its fresh and earthy taste while benefiting from its numerous health-boosting properties, knowing that you are doing something good for your body.

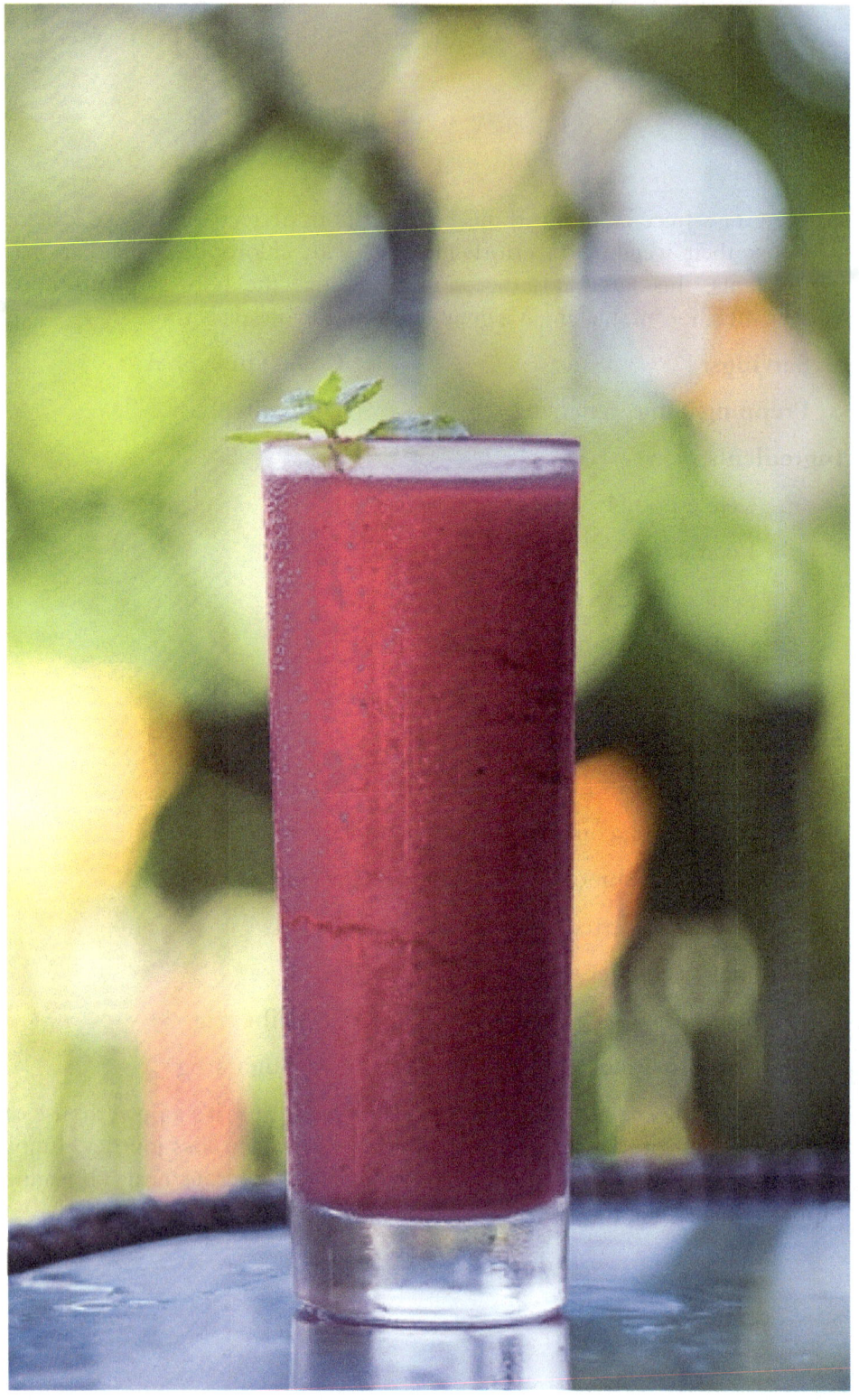

Cabbage & Pear Juice

Cabbage and pear Juice is not just a tasty blend, but also a powerful tool in your weight loss and detoxification journey. Packed with fiber, vitamins, and antioxidants, it is a great way to improve digestion and boost metabolism. The sweetness of pear perfectly balances the earthy taste of cabbage, making it a refreshing and healthy choice.

Servings: 1

Cook Time: N/A

Prepping Time: 5 minutes

Difficulty: Easy

Ingredients:

- ✓ 1 cup green cabbage, chopped
- ✓ 1 pear, cored and chopped
- ✓ ½ cucumber, peeled
- ✓ ½ lemon, juiced
- ✓ ½ cup water

Step-by-Step Preparation:

1. Wash and chop all ingredients.
2. Place cabbage, pear, cucumber, and lemon juice in a blender.
3. Add water and blend until smooth.
4. Strain the Juice if preferred and serve.

Nutritional Facts (Per serving):

- ❖ **Calories**: 50
- ❖ **Fiber**: 4g
- ❖ **Carbohydrates**: 12g
- ❖ **Sugars**: 8g

Cabbage & Pear Juice is an excellent addition to your weight loss journey. It is light, refreshing, and packed with nutrients that will keep you energized while supporting your body's natural detoxification process.

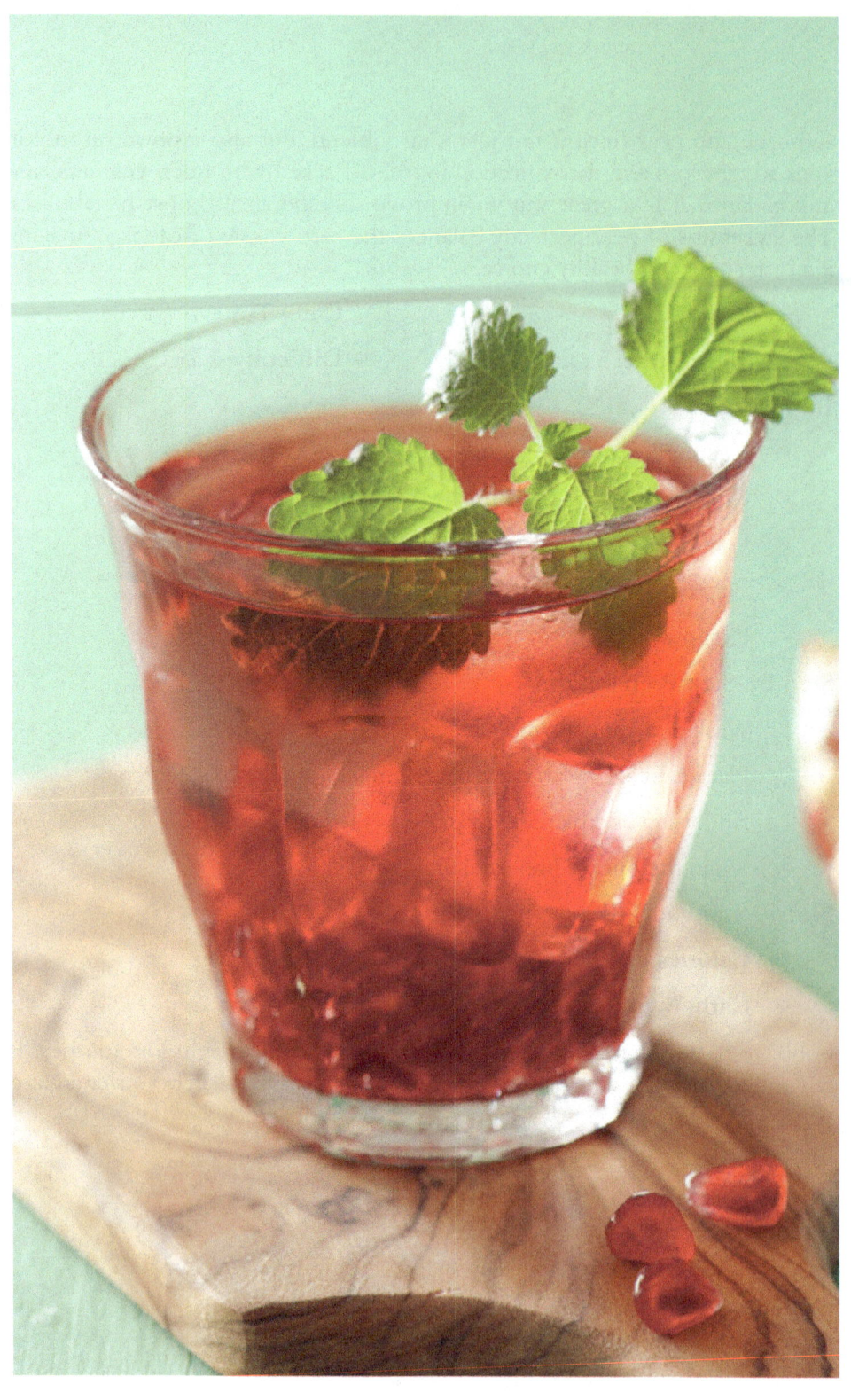

Pomegranate & Green Tea Detox Juice

Pomegranate & Green Tea Detox Juice is a delicious, antioxidant-rich drink promoting weight loss and boosting metabolism. The combination of fresh pomegranate juice and brewed green tea provides a burst of flavor while supporting detoxification and fat-burning processes in the body.

Servings: 1   **Cook Time**: N/A

Prepping Time: 5 minutes   **Difficulty**: Easy

Ingredients:

- ✓ ½ cup fresh pomegranate seeds
- ✓ 1 cup brewed green tea, cooled
- ✓ ½ lemon, juiced
- ✓ 1 teaspoon honey (optional)
- ✓ Ice cubes (optional)

Step-by-Step Preparation:

1. Brew green tea and let it cool.
2. Blend pomegranate seeds to extract juice.
3. Mix pomegranate juice, green tea, lemon juice, and honey (if using).
4. Stir well, add ice cubes if desired, and serve.

Nutritional Facts (Per serving):

- ❖ **Calories**: 45
- ❖ **Carbohydrates**: 10g
- ❖ **Fiber**: 1g
- ❖ **Sugars**: 8g

This Pomegranate & Green Tea Detox Juice is not just a refreshing beverage, but also a powerful tool in your health and wellness arsenal. Packed with health benefits, it helps cleanse the body, improve digestion, and support your weight loss journey. By incorporating this drink into your routine, you can feel reassured that you are taking a proactive step towards your health goals.

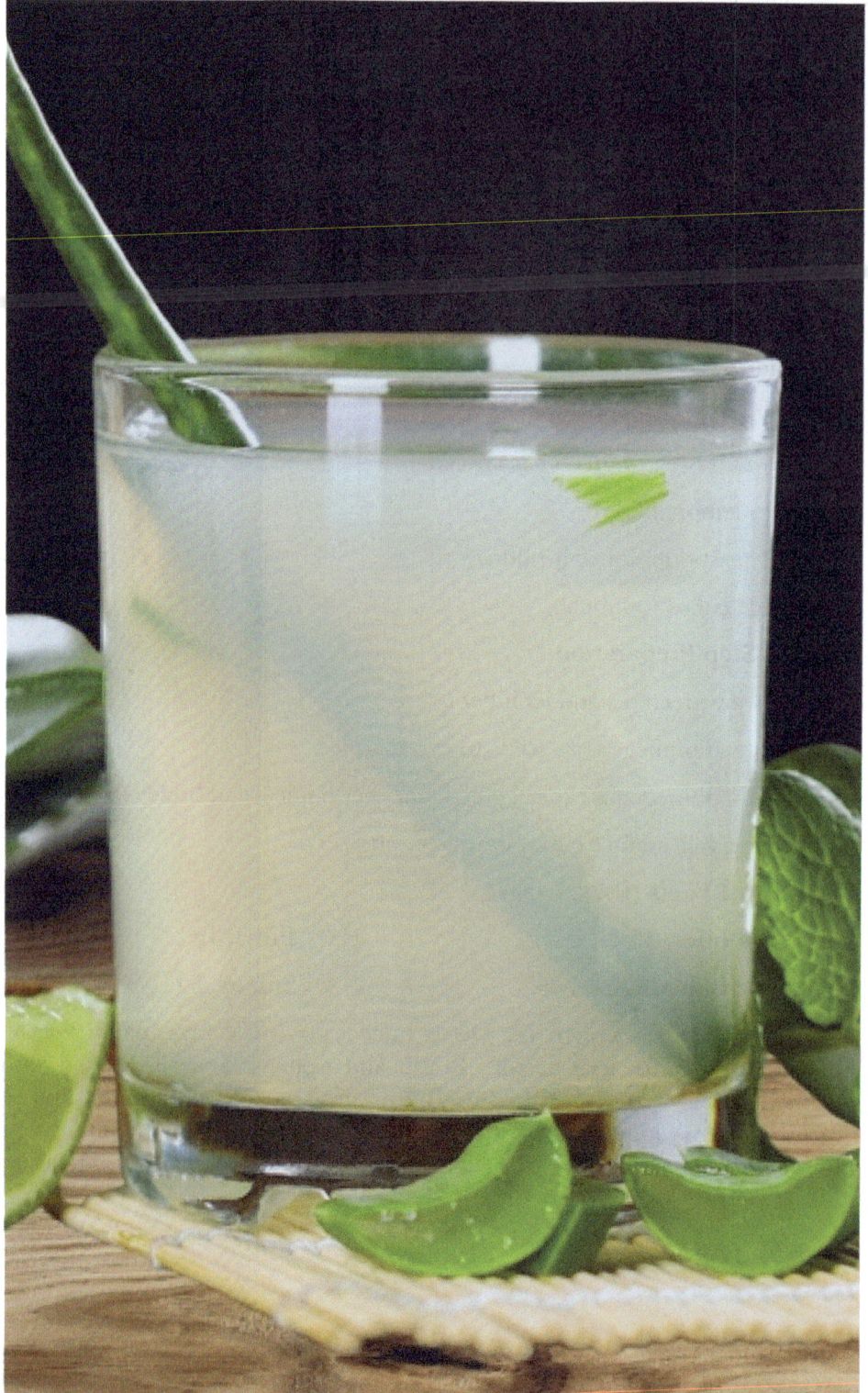

Aloe Vera & Lemon Juice

Aloe Vera & Lemon Juice is not just a refreshing and cleansing drink, but also a powerhouse of health benefits. Packed with vitamins, antioxidants, and hydrating properties, this juice aids in detoxifying your system, boosting metabolism, and enhancing fat-burning processes. Its effectiveness in promoting weight loss and boosting digestion makes it a perfect addition to your wellness routine, ensuring you are on the right track to a healthier you.

Servings: 1

Prepping Time: 5 minutes

Cook Time: N/A

Difficulty: Easy

Ingredients:

- ✓ 2 tablespoons fresh aloe vera gel
- ✓ 1 tablespoon lemon juice
- ✓ 1 cup water
- ✓ 1 teaspoon honey (optional)

Step-by-Step Preparation:

1. Extract fresh aloe vera gel from the leaf.
2. Mix aloe vera gel, lemon juice, and water in a glass.
3. Stir well and add honey if desired.
4. Serve chilled or at room temperature.

Nutritional Facts (Per serving):

- ❖ **Calories**: 15
- ❖ **Carbohydrates**: 4g
- ❖ **Sugars**: 2g
- ❖ **Vitamin C**: 10% DV

Aloe Vera & Lemon Juice is not just a drink, it's a natural and effective detox solution. It is a refreshing and cleansing drink that supports weight loss and keeps you feeling light and energized. With this hydrating beverage, you can trust that your body is getting the cleanse and refresh it needs daily, all from a natural and effective source.

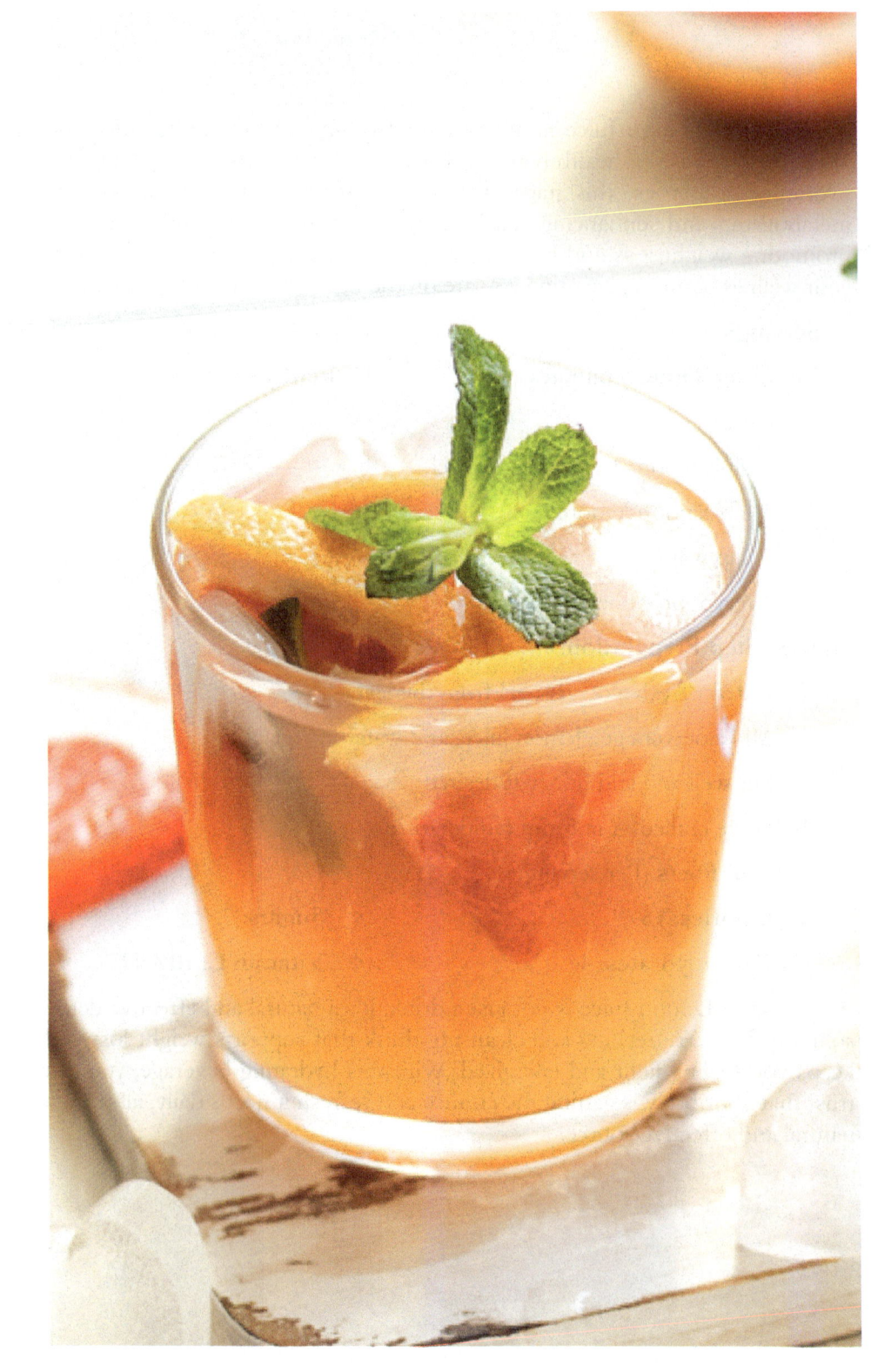

Grapefruit & Mint Detox Juice

This grapefruit & Mint Detox Juice is not just a refreshing and tangy beverage, it is a powerhouse of health benefits. Packed with antioxidants and vitamins, it is a great aid for weight loss. The combination of grapefruit and mint not only aids digestion but also promotes fat burning, making it a perfect addition to your wellness routine.

Servings: 1

Cook Time: N/A

Prepping Time: 5 minutes

Difficulty: Easy

Ingredients:

- ✓ 1 grapefruit, peeled and segmented
- ✓ 5-6 fresh mint leaves
- ✓ ½ lemon, juiced
- ✓ 1 teaspoon honey (optional)
- ✓ ½ cup water
- ✓ Ice cubes (optional)

Step-by-Step Preparation:

1. Peel and segment the grapefruit.
2. Blend the grapefruit, mint leaves, lemon juice, honey, and water.
3. Strain the juice if desired and pour over ice.
4. Serve chilled, and enjoy.

Nutritional Facts (Per serving):

- ❖ **Calories**: 50
- ❖ **Fiber**: 2g
- ❖ **Carbohydrates**: 12g
- ❖ **Sugars**: 9g

This Grapefruit and mint Detox Juice is a delicious, nutrient-packed drink that supports weight loss and keeps you feeling fresh and energized. Its detoxifying properties make it ideal for cleansing your body and enhancing your metabolism. For best results, consume this juice in the morning on an empty stomach.

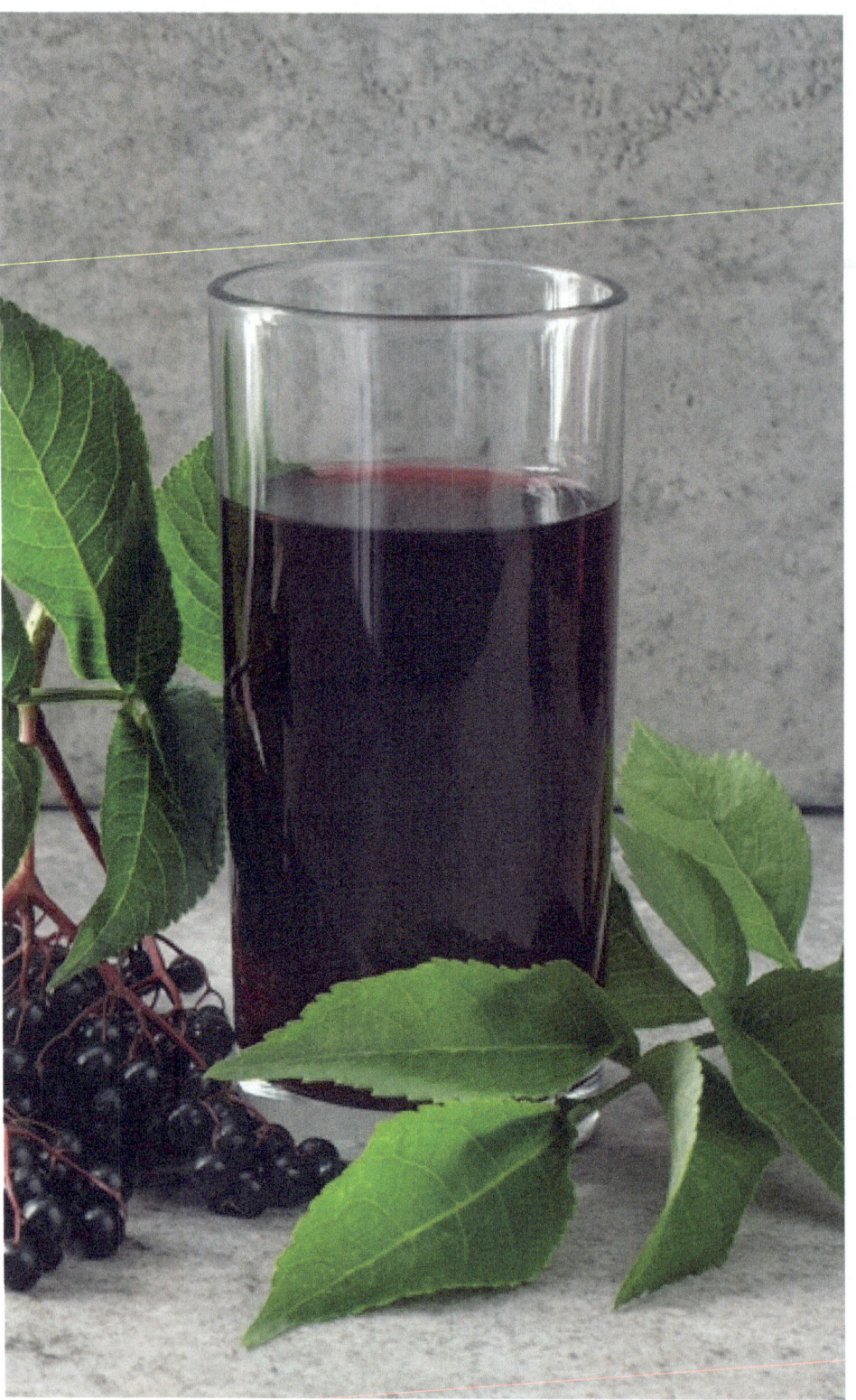

Immune Boosting Juices

Elderberry Immune Juice

This elderberry juice recipe, rich in antioxidants and essential nutrients, is not just a refreshing drink. It is a powerful tool to boost your immune system and promote weight loss. By adding this to your daily routine, you are making a proactive choice for your health. Imagine the benefits you will reap from this simple, yet powerful, addition to your diet.

Servings: 1

Prepping Time: 5 minutes

Cook Time: None

Difficulty: Easy

Ingredients:

- ✓ ½ cup elderberries (fresh or frozen)
- ✓ 1 apple, chopped
- ✓ 1 lemon, juiced
- ✓ ½ inch ginger root
- ✓ 1 cup water

Step-by-Step Preparation:

1. Rinse the elderberries and apples.
2. Add all ingredients to a blender.
3. Blend until smooth.
4. Strain the mixture for a smooth juice.
5. Serve chilled.

Nutritional Facts (Per serving):

- ❖ **Calories**: 85
- ❖ **Vitamin C**: 60% of Daily Value
- ❖ **Fiber**: 3g
- ❖ **Antioxidants**: High

Enjoy this delicious elderberry juice as part of a healthy, balanced diet to boost immunity, aid digestion, and naturally support your weight loss goals!

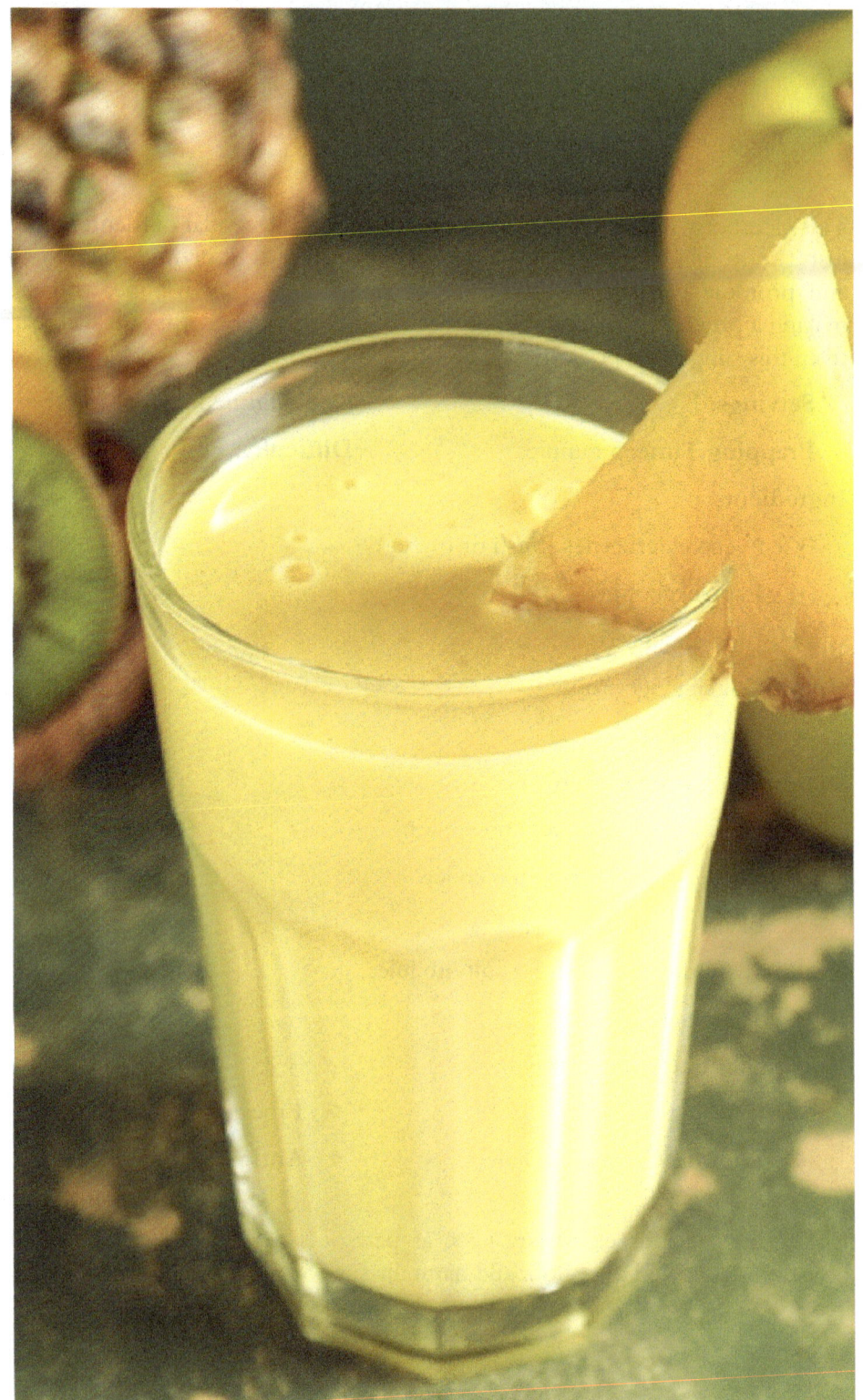

Vitamin C Booster

This Vitamin C Booster Juice is not just a delicious blend of pineapple, orange, and kiwi. It is a powerhouse of immune-boosting properties and a great aid for weight loss. Packed with antioxidants, this juice is a quick and easy way to add a healthy boost to your day, reassuring you that you are making a nutritious choice.

Servings: 1

Prepping Time: 5 minutes

Cook Time: None

Difficulty: Easy

Ingredients:

- ✓ ½ cup pineapple chunks
- ✓ 1 orange, peeled
- ✓ 1 kiwi, peeled
- ✓ ½ lemon, juiced
- ✓ ½ cup water

Step-by-Step Preparation:

1. Peel and chop the fruits.
2. Add all ingredients to a blender.
3. Blend until smooth.
4. Strain the juice for a smoother consistency.
5. Serve chilled, and enjoy.

Nutritional Facts (Per serving):

- ❖ **Calories**: 90
- ❖ **Vitamin C**: 150% of Daily Value
- ❖ **Fiber**: 4g
- ❖ **Antioxidants**: High

Sip on this revitalizing Vitamin C booster juice to fuel your weight loss journey while nourishing your body with essential vitamins and antioxidants!

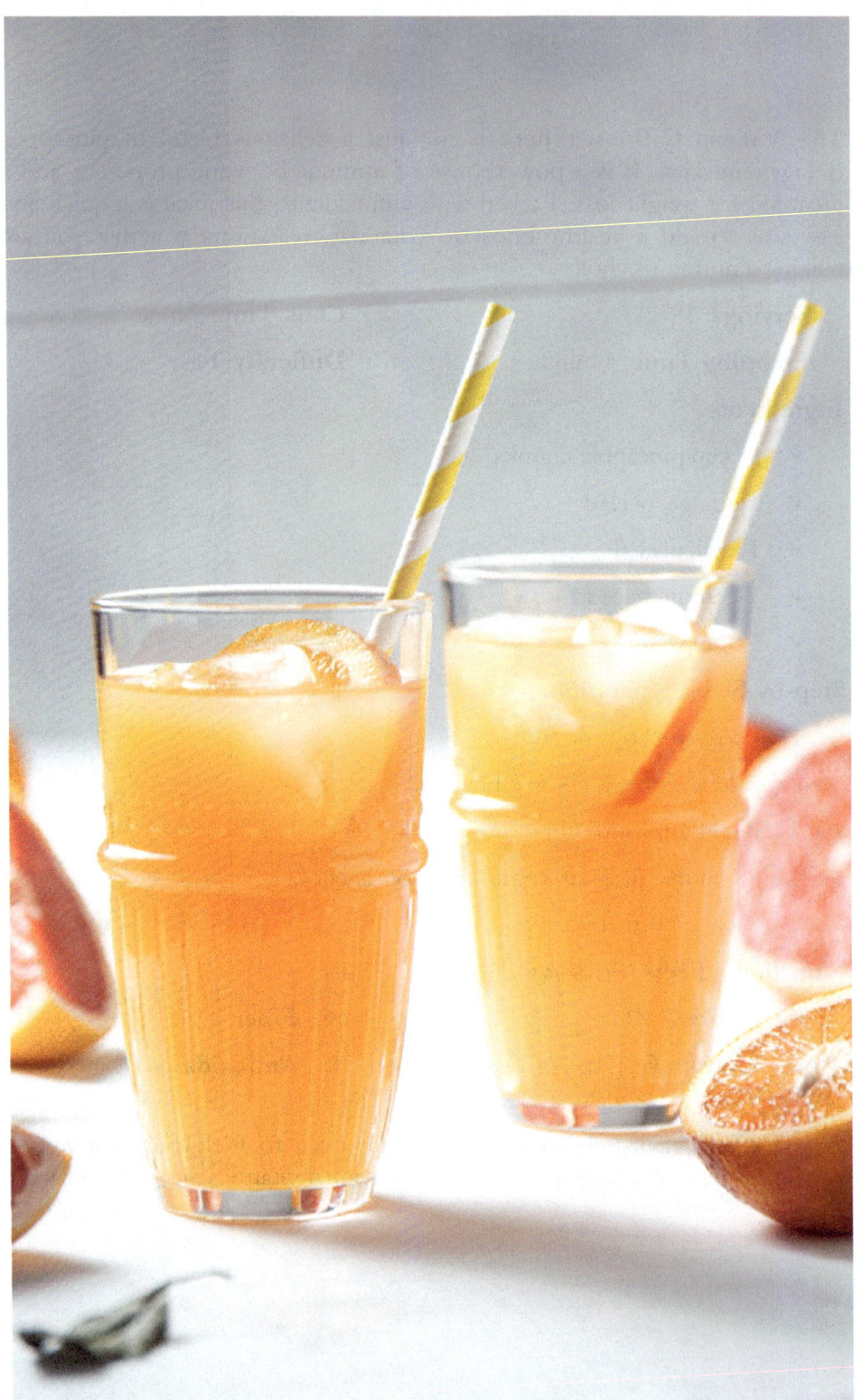

Citrus Immune Blast

The Citrus Immune Blast Juice is not just a delicious blend of orange, grapefruit, and lemon. It is a powerful tool in your quest for wellness. Packed with vitamin C and antioxidants, this refreshing juice is a potent boost to your immune system and a supportive ally in your weight loss journey.

Servings: 2

Cook Time: None

Prepping Time: 5 minutes

Difficulty: Easy

Ingredients:

- ✓ 2 oranges, peeled
- ✓ 1 grapefruit, peeled
- ✓ 1 lemon, juiced
- ✓ ½ cup water

Step-by-Step Preparation:

1. Peel and chop the oranges and grapefruit.
2. Add all ingredients, including lemon juice, into a blender.
3. Blend until smooth.
4. Strain the juice for a smoother texture.
5. Serve chilled, and enjoy.

Nutritional Facts (Per serving):

- ❖ **Calories**: 75
- ❖ **Fiber**: 3g
- ❖ **Vitamin C**: 130% of Daily Value
- ❖ **Antioxidants**: High

Sip this refreshing juice to stay hydrated, boost immunity, and naturally support your weight loss goals with the goodness of citrus fruits!

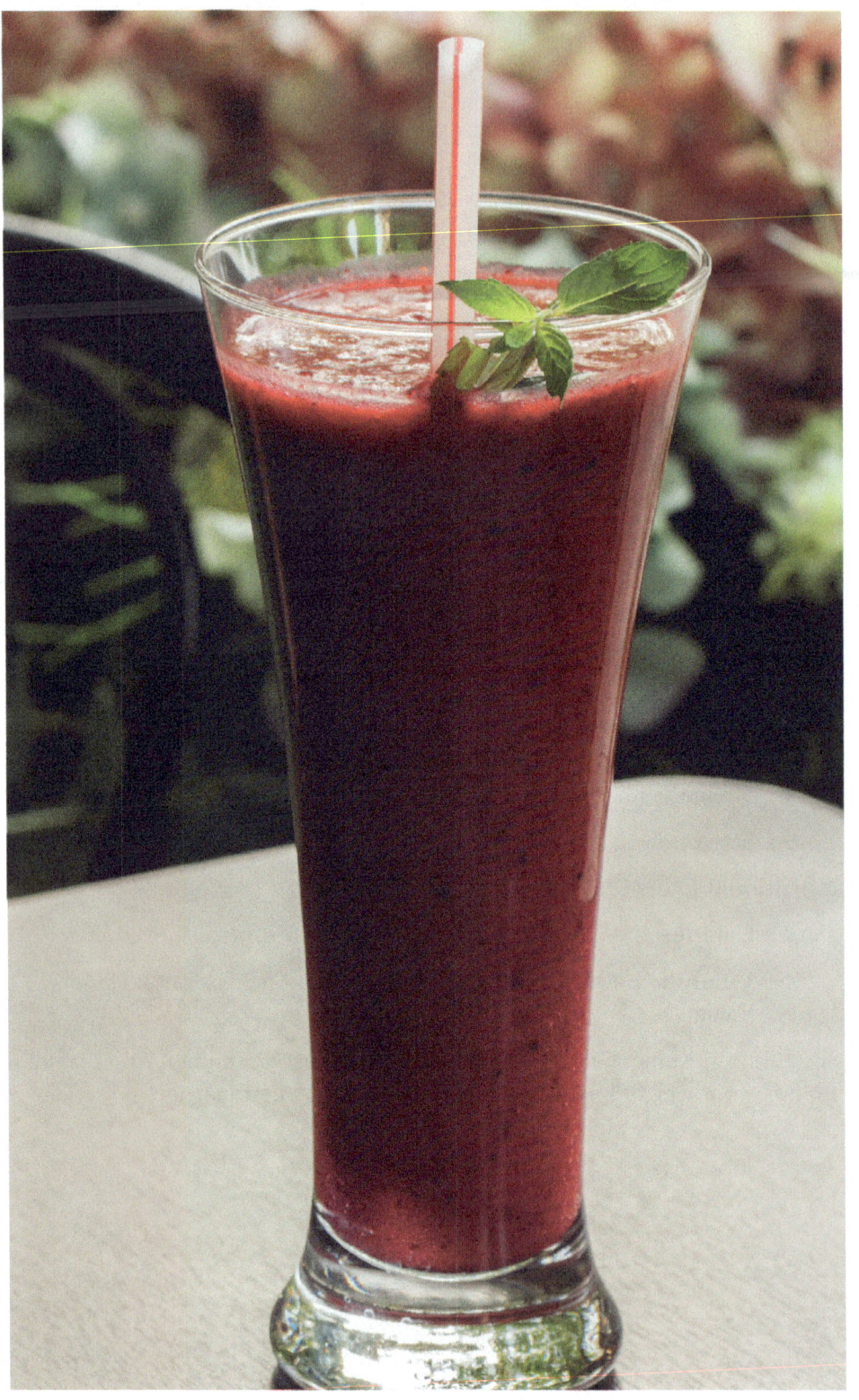

Berry Immune Elixir

The Berry Immune Elixir is not just a delicious blend of blueberry, raspberry, and fresh orange juice. It is a powerhouse of antioxidants and vitamin C, carefully crafted to boost your immune system and aid in weight loss. This nutrient-rich juice is a flavorful way to kickstart your day or refresh yourself post-workout, knowing that you are giving your body the best.

Servings: 1

Prepping Time: 5 minutes

Cook Time: None

Difficulty: Easy

Ingredients:

- ✓ ½ cup blueberries
- ✓ ½ cup raspberries
- ✓ 1 orange, juiced
- ✓ ½ cup water

Step-by-Step Preparation:

1. Rinse the berries thoroughly.
2. Add blueberries, raspberries, orange juice, and water into a blender.
3. Blend until smooth.
4. Strain the juice for a smoother consistency.
5. Serve chilled.

Nutritional Facts (Per serving):

- ❖ **Calories**: 95
- ❖ **Vitamin C**: 120% of Daily Value
- ❖ **Fiber**: 4g
- ❖ **Antioxidants**: High

Take a moment to savor this refreshing Berry Immune Elixir. Let its natural immune-boosting properties and the energy it provides be a treat for your body. With the power of berries, you can enjoy supporting your weight loss goals in a delightful way.

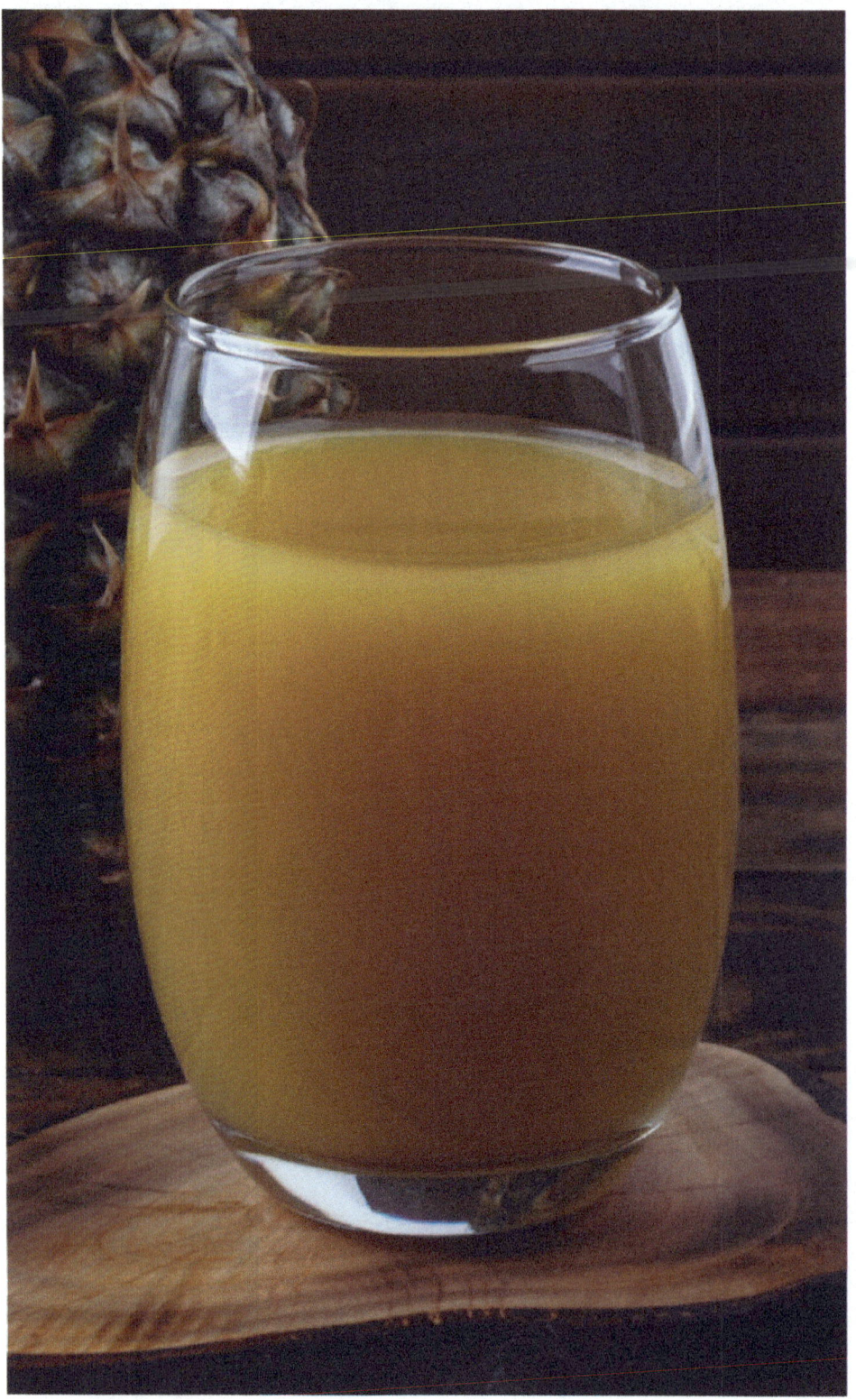

Anti-inflammation Immunity Boost

This Anti-inflammation Immunity Boost juice is not just a delicious drink; it is a powerful tool for your health. By combining the tropical sweetness of pineapple with the anti-inflammatory power of turmeric and ginger, this juice is packed with nutrients that can help reduce inflammation, strengthen your immune system, and aid in weight loss. It is a perfect addition to your healthy lifestyle, giving you the power to take control of your health.

Servings: 1

Prepping Time: 5 minutes

Cook Time: None

Difficulty: Easy

Ingredients:

- ✓ ½ cup pineapple chunks
- ✓ ½ inch fresh ginger root
- ✓ ½ tsp turmeric powder or fresh turmeric root
- ✓ ½ lemon, juiced
- ✓ ½ cup water

Step-by-Step Preparation:

1. Peel and chop the pineapple and ginger.
2. Add all ingredients to a blender.
3. Blend until smooth.
4. Strain the juice for a smoother texture.
5. Serve chilled, and enjoy.

Nutritional Facts (Per serving):

- ❖ **Calories**: 80
- ❖ **Vitamin C**: 90% of Daily Value
- ❖ **Fiber**: 2g
- ❖ **Anti-inflammatory**: High

This delicious and nutritious juice is a perfect way to combat inflammation, boost your immunity, and support weight loss while savoring the tropical flavors of pineapple and the warmth of turmeric and ginger. It offers a refreshing and tangy taste with a hint of warmth from the ginger and turmeric.

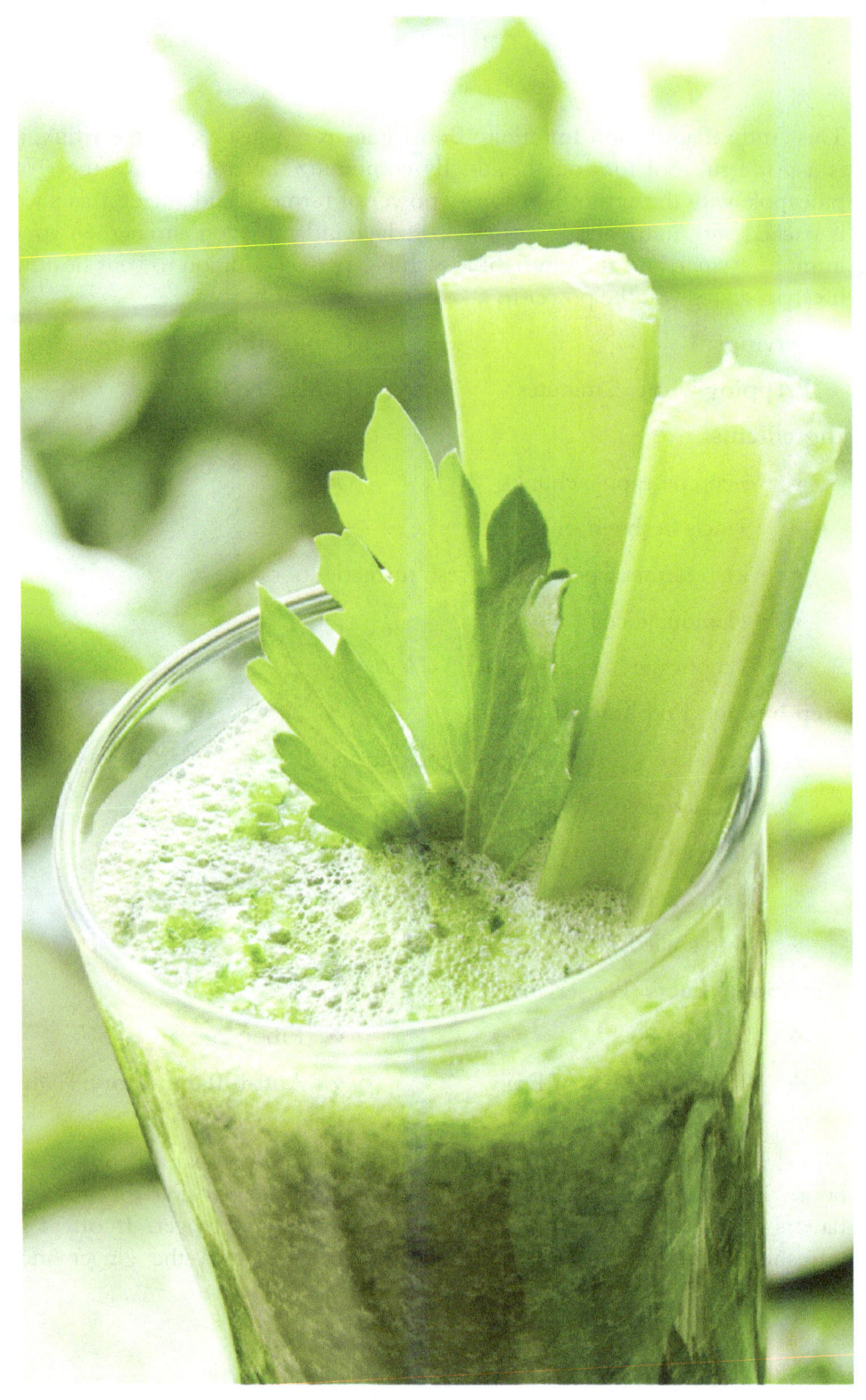

Anti-aging and Energizing Juices

Youthful Glow Juice

This Youthful Glow Juice is a refreshing blend of natural ingredients-cucumber, aloe vera, celery, and lemon. These ingredients are known for their hydrating, rejuvenating, and energizing properties. Packed with vitamins and antioxidants, this juice is a natural way to promote a youthful appearance and boost your energy levels.

Servings: 1

Prepping Time: 5 minutes

Cook Time: None

Difficulty: Easy

Ingredients:

- ✓ ½ cucumber, peeled
- ✓ 2 tbsp aloe vera gel (fresh or bottled)
- ✓ 1 celery stalk
- ✓ ½ lemon, juiced
- ✓ ½ cup water

Step-by-Step Preparation:

1. Peel and chop the cucumber and celery.
2. Add cucumber, celery, aloe vera, lemon juice, and water into a blender.
3. Blend until smooth.
4. Strain the juice for a smoother texture.
5. Serve chilled.

Nutritional Facts (Per serving):

- ❖ **Calories**: 45
- ❖ **Vitamin C**: 50% of Daily Value
- ❖ **Hydration**: High
- ❖ **Antioxidants**: Rich

Enjoy this revitalizing Youthful Glow Juice to nourish your skin, promote anti-aging benefits, and feel energized throughout the day. It contains the natural goodness of cucumber, aloe vera, and lemon!

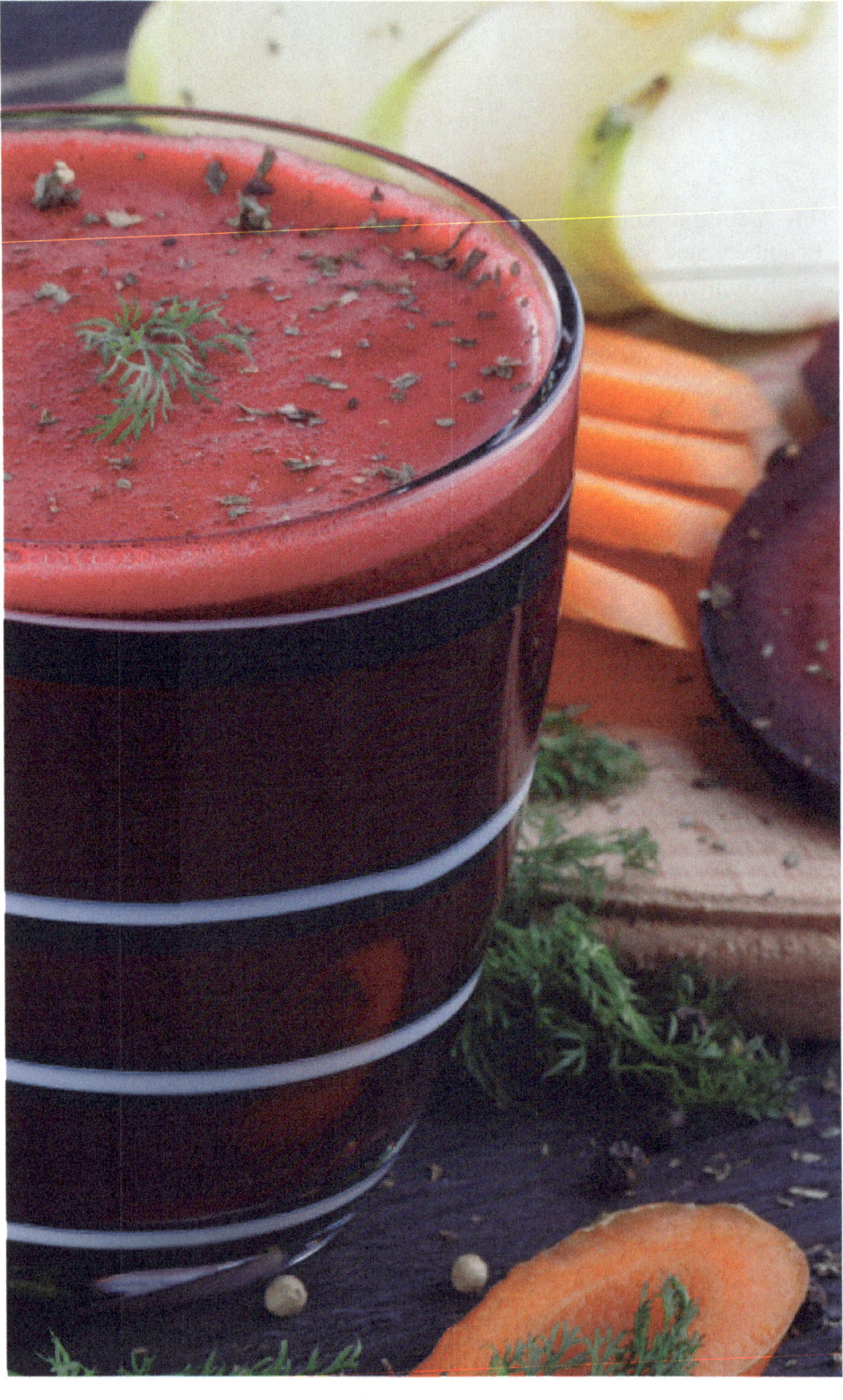

Anti-aging Powerhouse

This Anti-aging Powerhouse Juice is not just a delicious blend of beet, carrot, and apple. It is a rich source of vitamins and antioxidants that promote youthful skin and boost energy levels. By incorporating this nutrient-packed juice into your daily routine, you can be reassured that you are supporting healthy aging from the inside out.

Servings: 1

Prepping Time: 5 minutes

Cook Time: None

Difficulty: Easy

Ingredients:

- ✓ 1 small beet, peeled
- ✓ 1 carrot, peeled
- ✓ 1 apple, cored
- ✓ ½ lemon, juiced
- ✓ ½ cup water

Step-by-Step Preparation:

1. Peel and chop the beet, carrot, and apple.
2. Add all ingredients to a blender.
3. Blend until smooth.
4. Strain the juice for a smoother texture.
5. Serve chilled.

Nutritional Facts (Per serving):

- ❖ **Calories**: 90
- ❖ **Vitamin A**: 80% of Daily Value
- ❖ **Vitamin C**: 50% of Daily Value
- ❖ **Antioxidants**: Rich

So why not treat yourself to this energizing Anti-aging Powerhouse Juice? It is a delightful way to support glowing skin, reduce the signs of aging, and fuel your body with essential nutrients for a youthful, vibrant you!

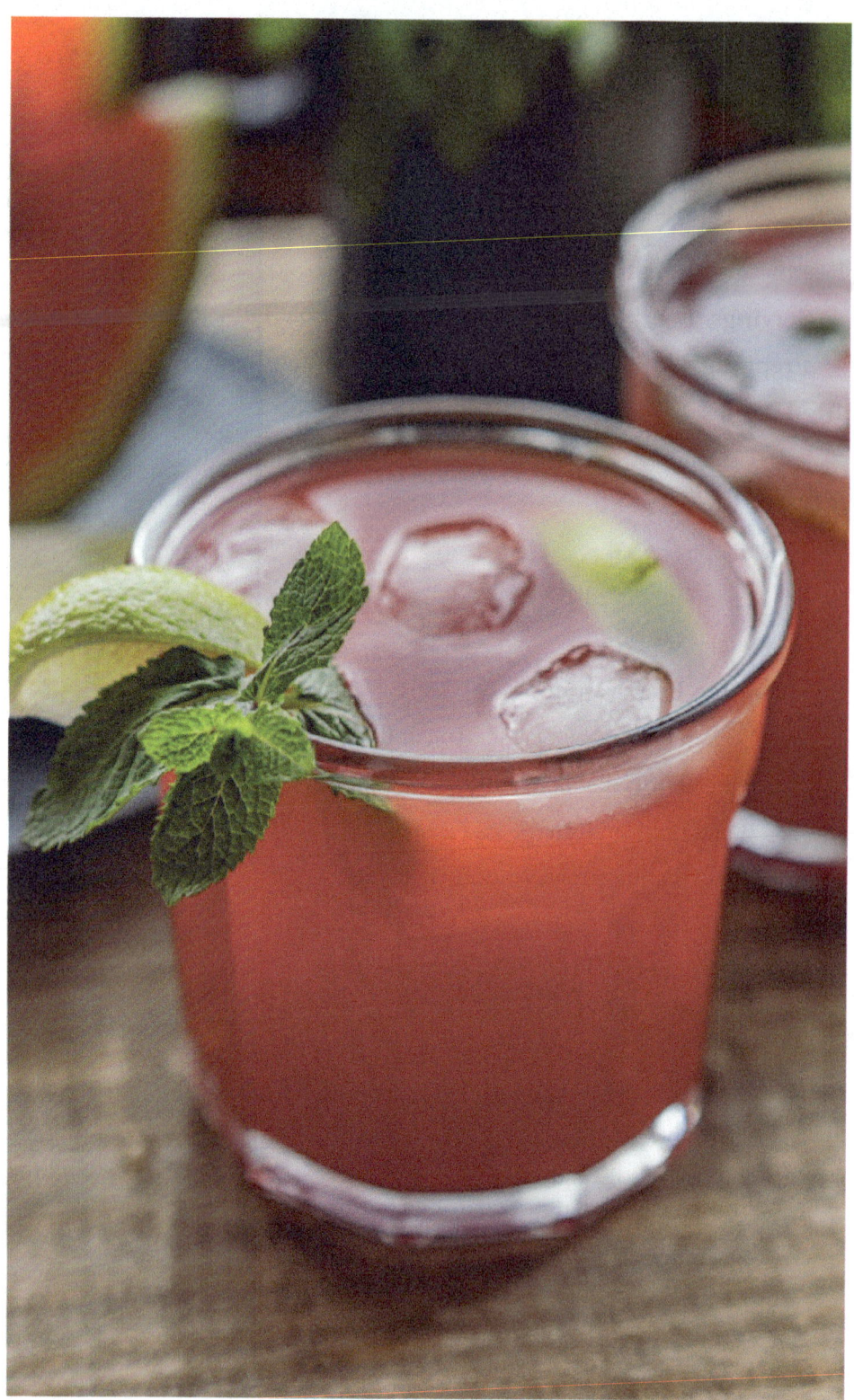

Vibrant Energy Juice

The Vibrant Energy Juice is a refreshing blend of watermelon, mint, and lime designed to hydrate, energize, and combat signs of aging. Rich in antioxidants and vitamins, this revitalizing drink is perfect for boosting energy levels and keeping skin glowing.

Servings: 2

Prepping Time: 5 minutes

Cook Time: None

Difficulty: Easy

Ingredients:

- ✓ 2 cups watermelon, chopped
- ✓ 10 fresh mint leaves
- ✓ 1 lime, juiced
- ✓ ½ cup water

Step-by-Step Preparation:

1. Chop the watermelon and rinse the mint leaves.
2. Add watermelon, mint, lime juice, and water into a blender.
3. Blend until smooth.
4. Strain for a smoother texture.
5. Serve chilled.

Nutritional Facts (Per serving):

- ❖ **Calories**: 60
- ❖ **Vitamin C**: 40% of Daily Value
- ❖ **Hydration**: High
- ❖ **Antioxidants**: Rich

So, next time you need a refreshing boost, reach for this Vibrant Energy Juice. It is not just a delicious drink, it is a way to stay hydrated, feel energized, and support youthful skin. It's refreshing combination of watermelon, mint, and lime will do the trick!

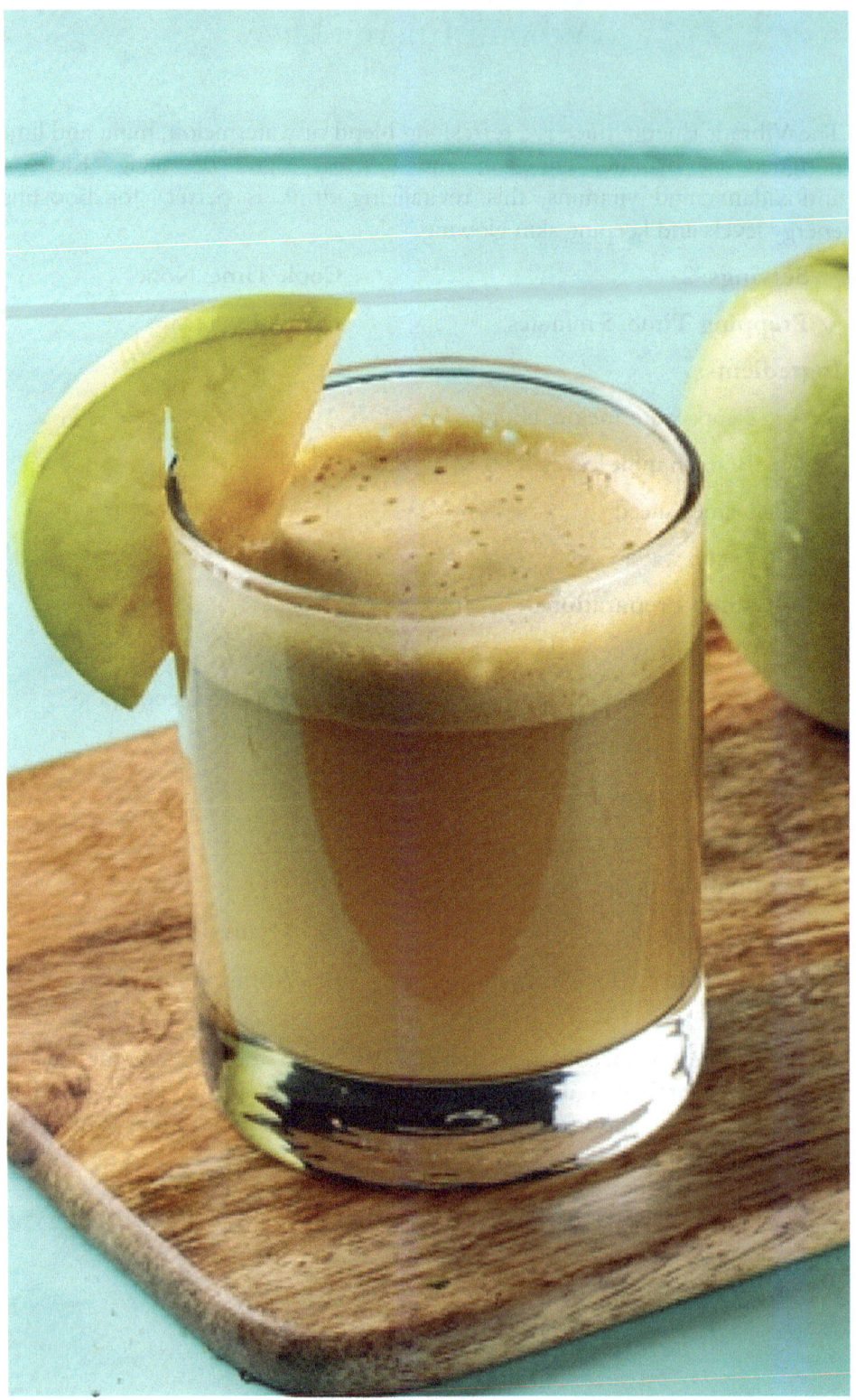

Apple-Ginger Radiance Booster

The Apple-Ginger Radiance Booster is not just a delicious blend of fresh apples and ginger, but also a powerhouse of health benefits. Packed with antioxidants and vitamin C, this juice is a natural energy booster and a potent anti-aging solution. By incorporating this into your routine, you can be reassured of its positive impact on your health and vitality.

Servings: 2

Prepping Time: 5 minutes

Cook Time: None

Difficulty: Easy

Ingredients:

- ✓ 2 apples, cored
- ✓ 1 inch fresh ginger root
- ✓ ½ lemon, juiced
- ✓ ½ cup water

Step-by-Step Preparation:

1. Core and chop the apples.
2. Peel and chop the ginger.
3. Add apples, ginger, lemon juice, and water to a blender.
4. Blend until smooth.
5. Strain the juice for a smoother texture and serve chilled.

Nutritional Facts (Per serving):

- ❖ **Calories**: 85
- ❖ **Vitamin C**: 30% of Daily Value
- ❖ **Fiber**: 3g
- ❖ **Antioxidants**: High

Enjoy this refreshing juice to energize your body and nourish your skin with natural, anti-aging ingredients for a radiant glow! The Apple-Ginger Radiance Booster has a crisp, tangy flavor that is sure to invigorate your taste buds.

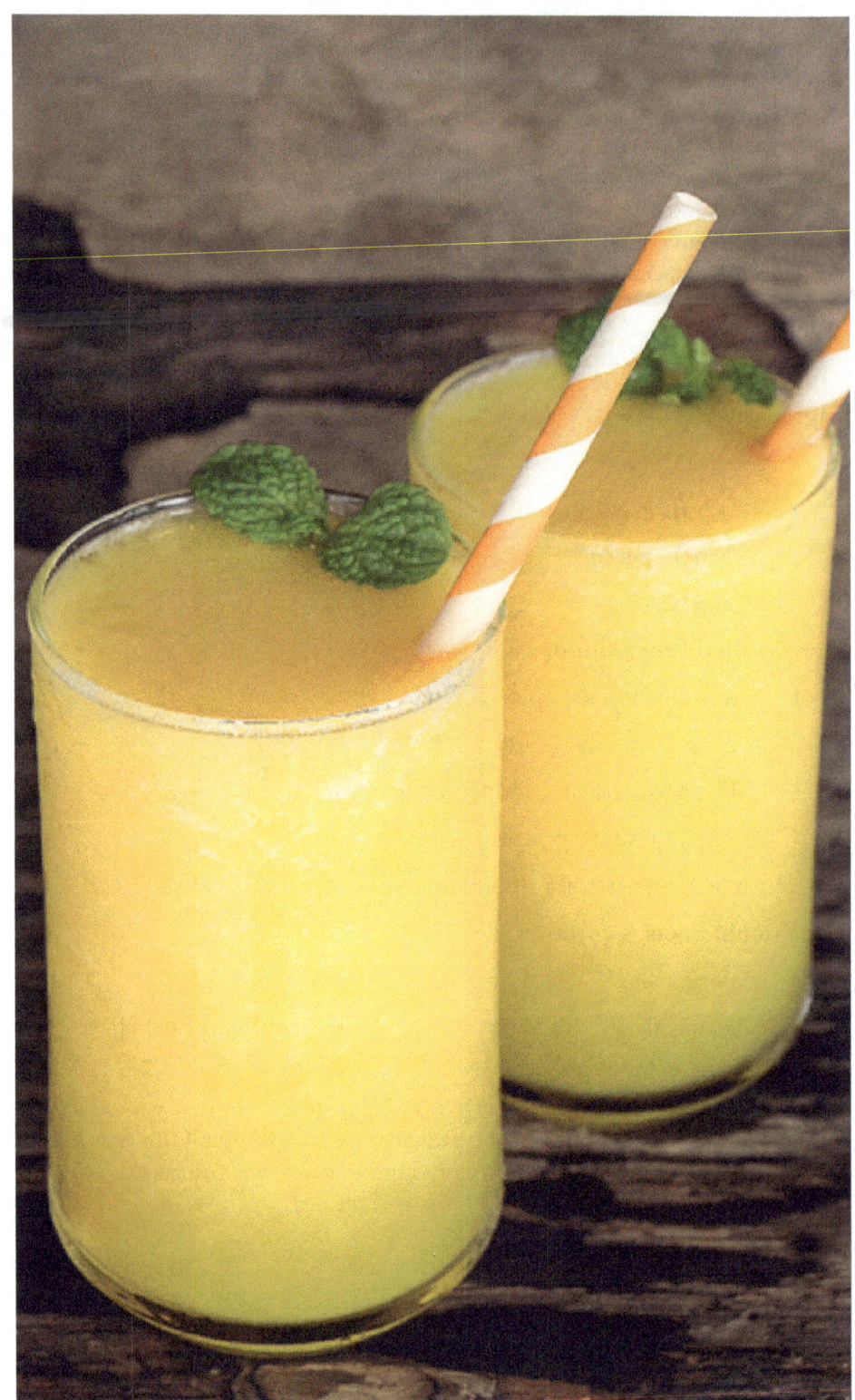

Mango-Orange Ageless Nectar

The Mango-Orange Ageless Nectar is a tropical blend of mango and orange. It is rich in vitamin C and antioxidants that support youthful skin and provide a natural energy boost. This refreshing juice helps fight signs of aging while energizing you throughout the day.

Servings: 2

Prepping Time: 5 minutes

Cook Time: None

Difficulty: Easy

Ingredients:

- ✓ 1 ripe mango, peeled and chopped
- ✓ 2 oranges, peeled
- ✓ ½ lemon, juiced
- ✓ ½ cup water

Step-by-Step Preparation:

1. Peel and chop the mango and oranges.
2. Add the mango, oranges, lemon juice, and water to a blender.
3. Blend until smooth.
4. Strain the juice for a smoother texture.
5. Serve chilled.

Nutritional Facts (Per serving):

- ❖ **Calories**: 120
- ❖ **Vitamin C**: 150% of Daily Value
- ❖ **Fiber**: 4g
- ❖ **Antioxidants**: High

This delicious Mango-Orange Ageless Nectar is the perfect blend of tropical flavors to keep your skin glowing and your energy levels high, offering a natural way to stay youthful and refreshed!

Conclusion

Achieving your weight loss goals does not have to be a challenge—juicing is a delicious, effective way to detox, energize, and melt fat while staying fit. In *Juicing Recipes for Weight Loss*, renowned nutritionist and juicing expert Clara Levine guides you through simple yet powerful juice recipes that you can easily incorporate into your daily routine. These recipes, backed by Clara's extensive knowledge and experience, help you shed pounds and boost your overall health and energy levels.

Are you ready to transform your body and revitalize your life? Imagine waking up each day feeling lighter, more energized, and confident in your weight loss journey. Whether you are a busy professional or just beginning your health journey, Clara's quick and easy juice-making guide is designed to fit into any lifestyle and give you the tools you need to achieve lasting results.

Take action now! If you have been searching for a simple solution to weight loss that works, now is the time to start juicing. Clara Levine's recipes are practical and enjoyable, packed with vibrant flavors and essential nutrients. You deserve a healthy body, and this guide makes achieving your weight loss goals more accessible.

Do not wait any longer. *Grab your copy of Juicing Recipes for Weight Loss today,* available in Kindle and Paperback. With Clara Levine's expert guidance, start your journey to detox, energize, melt fat, and stay fit. Your health transformation is just a juice away! Start your journey now by clicking the link below.

Made in the USA
Coppell, TX
20 June 2025

50965873R00066